YOUR FAMILY G
SYMPTOMS AND

YOUR FAMILY GUIDE TO SYMPTOMS AND TREATMENTS

DON R. POWELL, PhD

Edited by Dr Sue Davidson

Thorsons

An Imprint of HarperCollins*Publishers*

Thorsons
An Imprint of HarperCollins*Publishers*
77–85 Fulham Palace Road,
Hammersmith, London W6 8JB

Originally published as *The American
Institute for Preventive Medicine's Self-Care:
your family guide to symptoms and how to
treat them* 1996
This revised edition published by
Thorsons 1997
10 9 8 7 6 5 4 3 2 1

A catalogue record for this book
is available from the British Library

ISBN 0 7225 3370 5

Printed and bound in Great Britain
by Caledonian International Book
Manufacturing Ltd, Glasgow

CONTENTS

FOREWORD

Everyone who cares about their own or their family's health will find *Your Family Guide to Symptoms and Treatments* an invaluable addition to their personal health library. This handy book will help ensure that you and your family receive the health care you need – whether you can provide this care yourself, or whether you need to seek treatment from a doctor or other health professionals.

Your Family Guide to Symptoms and Treatments contains an abundance of information and practical advice that is both easy to find and simple to understand. The book has three main sections: Common Health Problems; Major Medical Conditions; and Emergency Procedures and Conditions.

Section 1: Common Health Problems This section forms the major part of the book. It covers the whole range of common health problems that you or members of your family are likely to encounter. Chapters within this section are devoted to problems affecting different parts of the body. There are also separate chapters on children's health, women's health and men's health.

For each common health problem, you will find a useful, jargon-free general description. This is followed by a 'Questions to Ask' flowchart, which has

been specially devised to help you make the right decisions about the type of action you should take. Should you seek emergency care? Should you see your doctor urgently? Should you make a non-urgent appointment with your doctor? Is it safe to treat yourself – and for how long? By helping you answer these questions, the easy-to-use flowcharts will help you take responsibility for your own health and for the health of your family. *Your Family Guide to Symptoms and Treatments* will also help you make best use of your doctor, seeing him or her only when it is necessary and being ready to provide the information that he or she needs.

Another major feature of this section is the wealth of information listed under the 'Self-Care Procedures' headings. You will find sound practical advice for the home treatment of every type of ailment. Where appropriate, you will also find advice on how to prevent a problem from recurring.

Section 2: Major Medical Conditions This section contains information on a wide range of major medical conditions. A general description of each condition is followed, where appropriate, by information on signs and symptoms, prevention, treatment and care. All the conditions included in this section need to be diagnosed by a doctor and treated by a health care professional. However, whenever possible, the book includes practical advice that you can follow to speed your recovery or help you feel more comfortable.

Section 3: Emergency Procedures and Conditions This short 'first aid' section will help you cope with medical emergencies and also with serious or common accidents of various kinds.

Your Family Guide to Symptoms and Treatments is not intended as a substitute for expert medical advice or treatment. The aim throughout is to help you to be better informed about health matters. You will then be able to make the best possible use of the various self-care and professional treatments available.

SECTION 1
COMMON HEALTH PROBLEMS

ABOUT THIS SECTION

You have to make a lot of decisions when you become ill, such as:

- Should I go to the nearest hospital with an Accident and Emergency Department?
- Should I call my doctor?
- Can I wait and see if it gets better?
- Can I take care of it myself?
- What self-treatments should I perform?

This section of *Your Family Guide to Symptoms and Treatments* can help answer these and other important questions. Detailed in this section are 91 common health problems and what you can do when you have one of them.

Sometimes you can treat these problems with self-care. Sometimes you need medical help. *Your Family Guide to Symptoms and Treatments* can help you ask the right questions and find the answers to take care of your health.

Each health problem discussed in this section is divided into three parts:

- Facts about the problem: What it is, what causes it, symptoms and treatments
- Yes and no questions to help you decide if you should get help fast, call your doctor, see your doctor or provide self-care
- A list of Self-Care Procedures for the problem

HOW TO USE THIS SECTION

- Find the problem in the table of contents in the beginning of the book and go to that page. The problems are listed in alphabetical order
- Read about the problem, what causes it (if known), its symptoms and treatments
- Ask yourself the 'Questions to Ask'. Start at the top of the flow chart and answer yes or no to each question. Follow the arrows until you get to one of these answers:

Seek Emergency Care

See Doctor

Call Doctor

Provide Self-Care

WHAT THE INSTRUCTIONS MEAN

Seek Emergency Care

You should get help fast. Go to the nearest hospital with an Accident and Emergency Department. Phone 999 for an emergency ambulance.

See Doctor

Note that the term doctor has been used in this book to refer to various members of the primary health care team based at your practice. These include:
- Your GP
- Practice nurse
- Midwife
- District nurse

When you see the 'See Doctor' symbol, you should do so as soon as you can. You may need medicine or treatment to keep the problem from getting worse. Call first and ask for an appointment or for a home visit. Tell the nurse or receptionist what's wrong if you can't talk to your doctor directly. If you can't be seen soon, ask whether you should go to an Accident and Emergency Department.

Call Doctor

Call your doctor and state the problem. He or she can decide what you should do. He or she may:

- Tell you to make an appointment to be seen
- Arrange to leave a prescription for you to collect
- Give you specific instructions to treat the problem

Provide Self-Care

You can probably take care of the problem yourself if you answered no to all the questions. Use the Self-Care Procedures that are listed. But call your doctor if your problem gets worse or the symptoms change. You may have some other problem.

CHAPTER 1
EYE, EAR, NOSE AND THROAT PROBLEMS

CONJUNCTIVITIS

Also known as sticky eye, red eye or pink eye, conjunctivitis is an inflammation of the conjunctiva, the underside of both the upper and lower eyelids and the covering of the white portion of the eye. The medical term for this is conjunctivitis. Some causes of conjunctivitis along with possible solutions are:

- Allergic reaction to airborne pollens, dust, mould spores and animal dander (flakes of dead skin) or direct contact with chlorinated water or cosmetics. If you can't avoid the allergens, antihistamines can help. So can certain eye drops. Ask your doctor which one(s) to use.
- Bacterial conjunctivitis (noted by a pus-like discharge). Warm compresses, along with an antibiotic ointment or prescription drops, can help. When treated correctly, bacterial conjunctivitis will clear up in two to three days, but you should continue to use the medicine as prescribed by your doctor.
- Viral conjunctivitis is a complication of a cold or flu. This type causes less discharge but more watering of the eyes than the bacterial form. Antibiotics don't work. Viral conjunctivitis can take 14 to 21 days to clear up.

Questions to Ask

Do you have severe eye pain or are your eyes sensitive to light? **YES**

 NO

Do you have a pus-like discharge that is yellowish-green in colour? **YES**

 NO

Have you tried the Self-Care Procedures listed but show no improvement after 24 hours, or have the symptoms worsened? **YES**

 NO

Self-Care Procedures

Here are some ways to relieve the symptoms of conjunctivitis:

- Don't touch the eye area with your fingers. If you must wipe your eyes, use tissues.
- With your eyes closed, apply a paper towel soaked in warm (not hot) water

to the affected eye three to four times a day for at least five minutes at a time. (These soaks also help to dissolve the crusty residue of conjunctivitis.)

- Use over-the-counter eye drops. They may soothe irritation and help relieve itching.
- Avoid wearing eye make-up until the infection has completely cleared up. (And never share make-up with others.)
- Don't cover or patch the eye. This can make the infection worse.
- Don't wear contact lenses while your eyes are infected.
- Wash your hands often and use your own towels. Conjunctivitis is very contagious and can be spread from one person to another by contaminated fingers, face cloths or towels.

EARACHE

Earaches can be slight or very painful. They are a sign that something is wrong. The most common cause of an earache is blocked eustachian tubes. These tubes go from the back of the throat to your middle ear. When eustachian tubes get blocked, fluid gathers, causing pain. Things that make this happen include an infection of the middle ear, colds, sinus infections and allergies. Other things that can cause ear pain include changes in air pressure in a plane, something stuck in the ear, too much ear wax, tooth problems and ear injuries.

Very bad earache should be treated by a doctor. Treatment will depend on its cause. Most often this includes pain relievers,

antibiotics (if infection is involved), methods to dry up or clear the blocked ear canal, and whatever else is necessary to treat the source of the pain. You can, however, use Self-Care Procedures if earache is slight and produces no other symptoms. One example is with a mild case of 'swimmer's ear', which affects the outer ear (see Self-Care Procedures).

Prevention

Much can be done to prevent earaches. Heed the old saying 'Never put anything smaller than your elbow into your ear.' This includes cotton buds, hair-grips, your fingers, etc. Doing so could damage your eardrum. When you blow your nose, do so gently, one nostril at a time. Don't smoke. Smoking and second-hand smoke can increase the risk of infection for you and persons around you, especially if they are prone to ear infections.

Questions to Ask

With the earache do you also have these symptoms:
- Stiff neck
- Fever
- Drowsiness
- Nausea, vomiting

YES

 NO

flowchart continued on next page

Did the pain start after a blow to the ear or recent head injury? **YES**

NO

Are any of these things present in an infant or small child especially following an upper respiratory infection, a cold, air travel or in a child with a history of ear problems:

- Constant pulling, touching or tugging at one or both ears
- Fever
- Constant crying despite being comforted
- Ear or ears that are hot and sensitive to the touch
- Unresponsiveness to loud noises, a bell or to the sound of your voice
- Irritability and sleeplessness especially at night or when lying down

YES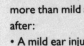

With the earache, do you also have hearing loss, ringing in the ears, dizziness or nausea? **YES**

NO

flowchart continued in next column

- Are there signs of infection such as:
- Fever (especially 38.5°C/101°F or higher)
- Discharge from the ear
- Severe ear pain and/or increased pain when wiggling the earlobe

YES

NO

Is the earache persistent, more than mild and occur after:

- A mild ear injury
- Hard or repeated nose blowings
- Sticking an object of any kind in the ear
- A cold, or sinus or upper respiratory infection
- Swimming, and is *extremely painful* when the earlobe is wiggled or touched
- Exposure to extremely loud noises (e.g., rock concerts, heavy machinery)

YES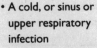

NO

Has a small object or insect entered the ear that cannot be easily or safely removed? **YES**

NO

flowchart continued on next page

Does the earache occur with jaw pain, headache or a clicking sound when opening and closing the mouth? **YES**

NO

Self-Care Procedures

To reduce pain:
- Place a warm face cloth or heating pad or wrapped hot water bottle next to the ear. Some health professionals recommend putting an ice bag or ice in a wet facecloth over the painful ear for 20 minutes.
- Take paracetamol, aspirin or ibuprofen. *Note: Do not give aspirin, or any medication containing salicylates, to children under 12 years of age, unless directed by a doctor, due to its association with Reye's syndrome, a potentially fatal condition.*

To open up the eustachian tubes and help them drain:
- Sit up.
- Prop your head up when you sleep.
- Yawn. (This helps move the muscles that open the eustachian tubes.)
- Chew gum or suck on a sweet. This is especially helpful during pressure changes that take place during air travel, but can also be useful during the middle of the night if you wake up with earache.
- Stay awake during takeoffs and landings when travelling by air.

- Take an oral decongestant such as pseudoephedrine (Sudafed), which can dry up the fluid in the ear that causes the pain. Decongestant nasal sprays can be used, but only for up to three days or as directed by your doctor. Take a decongestant:
  At the first sign of a cold if you have often had ear infections after previous colds
  One hour before you land when you travel by air if you have a cold or know your sinuses are going to block up
- Take a steamy shower.
- Have a steam inhalation.
- Use a room humidifier (or improvise with a wet towel over a radiator)
- Drink plenty of cool water.
- Gently, but firmly, blow through your nose while holding both nostrils closed until you hear a pop. This will help promote ear drainage and can be done several times a day.
- Feed a baby his or her bottle in an upright position, not with the child lying down.

In treating a mild case of swimmer's ear, the goal is to clean and dry the ear outer canal without doing further damage to the top layer of skin. What you can do:
- Shake your head to expel trapped water after swimming or showering.
- Hold your hand over your outer ear while tipping your head to that side.
- Do not remove earwax. This coats the ear canal and protects it from moisture. To avoid getting swimmer's ear:
- Wear wax or silicone earplugs that can be softened and shaped to fit your ears.

They are available at most chemists.
- Wear a bathing cap to help keep water from getting into your ears.
- Don't swim in dirty water.
- Swim on the surface of the water instead of beneath it.

EYESTRAIN FROM COMPUTER

Office workers have their share of work-related hazards. People who use visual display units (VDUs) may often complain of eyestrain, pain, stiffness in their backs and shoulders, and stress. These complaints can be a result of:

- Using a VDU for long periods
- Improper positioning of the VDU
- Poor lighting
- Poor posture
- Tight deadlines

VDU users can protect themselves from the physical problems that go with using them with the Self-Care Procedures listed.

Questions to Ask

Do you still have eyestrain, pain and stiffness in back and shoulders despite using Self-Care Procedures listed? **YES**

NO

Self-Care Procedures

To prevent eyestrain:
- Reduce glare. Keep the VDU away from windows. Turn off or shield overhead lights. Use a glare-reducing filter over the screen. Wear clothes that won't make you a source of glare.
- Place your paperwork close enough that you don't have to keep refocusing when switching from the screen to the paper. Use a paper holder.
- Place the screen so that your line of sight is 10 to 15 degrees (about one-third of a 45-degree angle) below horizontal.
- Dust off the screen often.
- Blink often to keep your eyes from getting dry. Use 'artificial tear' eyedrops if needed.
- Tell your optician that you use a VDU. Glasses and contact lenses worn for other activities may not be good for work on a VDU. (With bifocals, the near vision part of the lens is good for looking down, as when you read, but not straight ahead, as you do when looking at a visual display screen. So you may need single-vision lenses for VDU work.)
- If the image on the VDU screen is blurred, dull or flickering, have the screen serviced right away.
- Try to keep the VDU screen 60 cm (2 ft) away from your eyes.

To prevent muscle tension when you work on a VDU:
- Use a chair that supports your back and can be easily adjusted to a height that feels right for you.

- Take a 15-minute break if you can, for every two hours you use a VDU. Get up and go for a short walk, for example.
- Do stretching exercises of the neck, shoulder and lower back every one to two hours.
  - Rotate your head in a circular motion, first clockwise, then anti-clockwise.
  - Shrug your shoulders up and down, and backwards and forwards.
  - While standing or sitting, bend at the waist, leaning first to the left, then to the right.

HAY FEVER

Despite its name, hay fever has nothing to do with hay or fever. A nineteenth-century doctor called it this because he began to sneeze every time he entered a hay barn. But hay fever is, in fact, a reaction of the upper respiratory tract to anything to which you may be allergic. The medical terms for hay fever are seasonal rhinitis and perennial rhinitis. Symptoms include itchy, watery eyes; runny, itchy nose; congestion and sneezing. Hay fever is most common in spring and fall, but some people have it all year. You can try to avoid things that give you hay fever. Talk to your doctor if that doesn't help. He or she may prescribe antihistamines or nasal sprays. Here are a few tips on these medications:

- Antihistamines stop your body from making histamine, a substance your body makes when you are exposed to an allergen. Histamine causes many allergic symptoms. For best results, take the antihistamine 30 minutes before going outside. *Note: Some over-the-counter antihistamines may cause more drowsiness than prescription ones. Also, in case of drowsiness, care should be taken when driving and operating machinery. Antihistamines should be avoided during pregnancy.*
- Decongestants shrink the blood vessels in your nose and do not usually cause drowsiness.
- Nasal sprays containing steroids or cromolyn sodium are now available over the counter. They take several days to become effective and must be used regularly.

If your hay fever is very bad, your doctor may suggest allergy injections. First, you will be given skin tests to find out what causes your allergy. Then, over a period of several weeks, you will be given injections containing increasing amounts of allergen. These injections will reduce your body's sensitivity to the allergen.

Questions to Ask

Is it so hard for you to breathe that you can't talk (say four to five words between breaths)?  YES

NO

flowchart continued on next page

Do you have severe breathing difficulties or wheezing? **YES**	

Do you have symptoms of an infection such as fever, thick and discoloured nasal discharge or sputum, headache or muscle aches? **YES**	

Do you still have hay fever symptoms when you avoid hay fever triggers? **YES**	

Are hay fever symptoms interfering with your daily activities? **YES**	

NO

Self-Care Procedures

- Try to stay away from things that give you hay fever: Let someone else do outside chores. Mowing the lawn or raking leaves can make you very ill if you are allergic to pollen from grains, trees or weeds. It's a problem if you are allergic to moulds, too.
- Keep windows and doors shut and stay inside when the pollen count or humidity is high. Early morning is sometimes the worst.
- Try to keep dust, mould and pollen away from you at home and work:

- Dust and vacuum your home often.
- Wash rugs.
- Take carpets and curtains out of your bedroom.
- Cover your mattress with a plastic cover.
- Do not use a feather pillow.
- Stay away from stuffed animals. They collect dust.
- Don't have pets. If you must, keep them outside the house.
- Don't hang sheets and blankets outside to dry. Pollen can get on them.
- Shower, bathe and wash your hair following heavy exposure to pollens, dust, etc.
- Avoid tobacco smoke and other air pollutants.

HEARING LOSS

Do people seem to mumble a lot lately? Do you have trouble hearing in church or theatres? Is it hard to pick up what others say at the dinner table or at family gatherings? Does your family ask you to turn down the volume on the TV or radio?

These are signs of gradual, age-related hearing loss called presbycusis. High-pitched sounds are the ones to go first. Hearing loss from presbycusis cannot be restored, but hearing aids, along with the Self-Care Procedures listed, can be helpful.

Hearing loss can also result from other things:
- A blow to the ear
- Exposure to excessive noise including that generated by low-flying aircraft or types of heavy, loud machinery

- Blood vessel disorders including high blood pressure
- A blood clot that travels to nerves in the ear
- Ear wax that blocks the ear canal
- Chronic middle-ear infections or an infection of the inner ear
- Meniere's disease (a disease marked by excess fluid in the canals of the inner ear)
- Multiple sclerosis
- Syphilis
- Brain tumour

Babies and young children should have their hearing checked during routine developmental screening checks. You may suspect a hearing problem in your child if he or she isn't properly responding to sounds. You may also notice that he or she is not learning to speak as quickly as expected. Children can be born with hearing loss or develop it from an ear infection or upper respiratory infection.

Questions to Ask

In a child: Does the child not respond to any sound, even a whistle or loud clap? Did the child's mother have rubella (German measles) when pregnant with the child? Does the child not respond to sounds after:
- Recent earache or upper respiratory infection
- Air travel

YES

NO

In a child or adult: Do you have any of the following with the hearing loss:
- Discharge from the ear
- Earache
- Dizziness or feeling that things are spinning around you
- Recent ear or upper respiratory infection
- Feeling that the ears are blocked or filled with wax

YES

NO

Can you not hear the ticking of a ticking watch held next to the ear?

YES

NO

Do you hear a ringing sound in one or both ears all of the time?

YES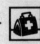

NO

Did you lose your hearing after being exposed to loud noises such as those associated with aircraft or work- or hobby-related loud noises (e.g., heavy machinery, power tools, firearms, etc.) and has this not improved?

YES

NO

Self-Care Procedures

For gradual, age-related hearing loss (presbycusis):
- Ask people to speak clearly, distinctly, and in a normal tone.
- Look at people when they are talking to you. Watch their expressions to help you understand what they are saying. Ask them to face you.
- Try to limit background noise when having a conversation.
- In a church or theatre, sit near the front.
- To rely on sight instead of sound, install a buzzer, flasher or amplifier on your telephone, door bell and alarm clock. Also, an audiologist (hearing therapist) may be able to show you other techniques for 'training' yourself to hear better.

To clear earwax: (Use only if you know that the eardrum is not perforated. Check with your doctor if you are in doubt.)
- Lie on your side. Using a syringe or medicine dropper, carefully squeeze a few drops of lukewarm water into your ear (or ask someone else to do this). Let the water stay there for 10 to 15 minutes and then shake it out.
- Do this again but use a few drops of olive oil or an over-the-counter cleaner such as Earex, Otex or Cerumol. Let the excess fluid flow out of the ear.
- After several minutes, follow the same procedure using warm water again, letting it remain there for 10 to 15 minutes. Tilt the head to allow it to drain out of the ear.

You can repeat this entire procedure again in three hours if the earwax has not cleared.

To prevent hearing loss:
- Don't put cotton buds, fingers, hair-grips, etc. in your ear.
- Don't blow your nose with too much force. It is better to blow your nose gently one nostril at a time with a tissue or handkerchief held loosely over the nostril.
- Avoid places that have loud noises (airports, construction sites, etc.). Protect your ears with earplugs.
- Keep the volume low on such items as personal stereos and car stereos. If someone else can hear the music when the earphones are on your head, the volume is too loud.
- Follow your doctor's advice for disorders that can cause hearing loss (e.g., high blood pressure, Meniere's disease, etc.).
- Avoid prolonged use of or overdosing on drugs that cause hearing loss (e.g., heavy use of aspirin or quinine).

Also be aware of things that can help you hear sounds if your hearing is impaired:
- Hearing aids. (See your GP.)
- Devices made to assist in hearing sounds from the TV and radio
- Special equipment that can be installed in your telephone by the telephone company
- Portable devices made especially to amplify sounds. (These can be used for classes, meetings, films etc.)

HICCUPS

Hiccups are simple enough to explain. Your diaphragm (the major muscle involved in breathing that sits like a cap over the stomach) goes into spasm. Things that promote hiccups are:

- Eating too fast, which causes you to swallow air along with food
- Eating fatty foods to the point where they make the stomach full enough to irritate the diaphragm

According to a doctor who studies hiccups, there is a hiccup centre in the brain that triggers a spasm of the esophagus setting in motion the cycle leading to hiccups. This, he thinks, is a protective mechanism to keep a person from choking on food or drink. Luckily, hiccups are generally harmless and don't last very long.

Questions to Ask

Do the hiccups occur with:
- Severe abdominal pain and
- Vomiting blood or blood in the stools

YES

NO

Have the hiccups lasted longer than eight hours in an adult or three hours in a child?

YES

NO

flowchart continued in next column

Have the hiccups started only after taking prescription medicine?

YES

NO

Self-Care Procedures

Luckily, there's no shortage of hiccup cures, and better still, most of them work (although some baffle medical science). A study reported in the *New England Journal of Medicine* found that one teaspoon of ordinary table sugar, swallowed dry, cured hiccups immediately in 19 out of 20 people (some of whom had been hiccuping for as long as six weeks). If this doesn't stop the hiccups right away, repeat it three times at two-minute intervals. Other popular folk remedies worth trying include:

- Hold your tongue with your thumb and index finger and gently pull it forward.
- With your neck bent back, hold your breath for a count of 10. Exhale immediately and drink a glass of water.
- Breathe into and out of a paper (not plastic) bag.
- Swallow a small amount of finely crushed ice.
- Massage the back of the roof of your mouth with a swab of cotton wool. A finger works equally well.
- Eat dry bread slowly.
- Drink a glass of water rapidly.

LARYNGITIS

Disc jockeys get laryngitis. So do actors, politicians and others who talk for hours. But ordinary people who overuse their voices get laryngitis, too. Perhaps you cheer too loudly and too often at a football match. Or perhaps you lose your voice for no apparent reason.

Air pollution or spending an evening in a smoky room can irritate the larynx (voice box) and cause laryngitis. Infections, too, can inflame the larynx. When your larynx is irritated or inflamed, your voice becomes hoarse, husky and weak. Sometimes laryngitis is painless, but you may get a sore throat, fever or dry cough, a tickling sensation in the back of the throat, or have trouble swallowing. Smoking, drinking alcohol, breathing cold air, and continuing to use already-distressed vocal cords can make the situation worse.

Questions to Ask

Is it hard for you to breathe or swallow or are you coughing up blood? **YES**

NO

Do you have a high fever or are you coughing up blood or yellowish-green sputum? **YES**

NO

flowchart continued in next column

Do you have hard, swollen lymph glands in your neck or do you feel like you have a 'lump in your throat'? **YES**

NO

Has the hoarseness lasted more than a week in a child or more than a month in an adult? **YES**

NO

Do you have two or more of these problems:
• Bothered by the cold more than usual
• Dry hair or skin
• Gaining weight for no reason
• Feeling very tired for no reason **YES**

NO

Self-Care Procedures

• Don't talk if you don't need to. Use a notepad and pencil to write notes instead. If you must speak, do so softly, but don't whisper.
• Drink lots of warm drinks. Tea with honey is good.
• Gargle with warm salt water ($^1/_4$ teaspoon of salt in $^1/_2$ cup of water).
• Take a hot shower or steam bath.

- Don't smoke. Stay away from places with smoky air.
- Suck on cough drops, throat lozenges or boiled sweets. (Do not give to children under age five.)
- Take aspirin, paracetamol or ibuprofen. *Note: Do not give aspirin, or any medication containing salicylates, to children under 12 years of age, unless directed by a doctor, due to its association with Reye's syndrome, a potentially fatal condition.*

NOSEBLEEDS

Nosebleeds are usually a childhood problem resulting from broken blood vessels just inside the nose. They're caused by a cold, frequent nose blowing and picking, allergies, a dry environment, using too much nasal spray, or a punch or other blow to the nose.

Not all nosebleeds are minor. Some are serious, such as heavy bleeding from deep within the nose (called a posterior nosebleed) that's hard to stop. This type usually strikes the elderly and is most commonly caused by hardening of nasal blood vessels, high blood pressure, drugs to treat blood clots, primary bleeding disorders like haemophilia, or by a tumour in the nose.

Questions to Ask

Did this nosebleed follow a blow to another part of the head?	YES	

NO

Does the nosebleed last 10 to 15 minutes or more?	YES	

NO

Does the nosebleed start after taking newly prescribed medication?	YES	

 NO

Do nosebleeds recur often and/or are they becoming more frequent?	YES	

 NO

Self-Care Procedures

Although there are lots of ideas about how to treat minor nosebleeds, the following procedure is recommended by the major first aid organizations.
- Sit with your head leaning forward.
- Pinch the nostrils shut, using your thumb and forefinger in such a way that the nasal septum (the nose's central partition) is being gently squeezed.
- Hold for 10 uninterrupted minutes, breathing through your mouth. Repeat if necessary.

- At the same time, apply cold compresses (such as ice in a soft cloth) to the area around the nose.
- Wait for four hours before blowing your nose, lifting heavy objects or exercising strenuously.
- For the next 24 hours, make sure your head is elevated above the level of your heart.

Note: If you are unable to stop a nosebleed by using the Self-Care Procedures, call your doctor.

SINUS PROBLEMS

Your sinuses are behind your cheekbones and forehead and around your eyes. Healthy sinuses drain over one litre (nearly two pints of water) every day. They keep the air you breathe wet. Your sinuses can't drain properly if they are infected and swollen. Your chances of getting a sinus infection increase if you:
- Have hay fever
- Smoke
- Have a nasal deformity or sinuses that don't drain well
- Have an abscess in an upper tooth
- Sneeze hard with your mouth closed or blow your nose too much when you have a cold
  Symptoms of a sinus infection are:
- Head congestion
- Nasal congestion and discharge (usually yellowish-green)
- Pain and tenderness over the facial sinuses
- Pain in the upper jaw

- Recurrent headache that changes with head position and disappears shortly after getting out of bed
- Fever

Sinus complications can be serious. Your doctor can sometimes tell if you have a sinus infection simply by examining you. In other cases he or she will also request a laboratory study of a sample of your nasal discharge and X-rays of the sinuses. You may need prescriptions for an antibiotic, a decongestant as well as a nasal spray and/or nose drops. These work to clear the infection and reduce congestion. (Severe cases may require surgery to drain the sinuses.)

Questions to Ask

Do you have two or more of the following:
- A fever over 38.5°C (101°F)
- Greenish-yellow or bloody-coloured nasal discharge
- A severe headache that doesn't get better when you take aspirin or paracetamol or that is worse in the morning or when you bend forwards
- Pain between the nose and lower eyelid
- A feeling of pressure inside the head

flowchart continued on next page

- Eye pain, blurred vision or changes in vision
- Pain in the cheek or upper jaw
- Swelling around the eyes, nose, cheeks and forehead
- Trouble sleeping or thinking clearly

YES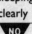

NO

Self-Care Procedures

A humidifier can help. Wet air helps make mucus thin. You can put a warm face cloth or compress on your face, too. This can help with the pain. Here are some more tips:

- Steam inhalations may help.
- Drink plenty of water and other liquids.
- Take aspirin, paracetamol or ibuprofen for pain. *Note: Do not give aspirin, or any medication containing salicylates, to children under 12 years of age, unless directed by a doctor, due to its association with Reye's syndrome, a potentially fatal condition.*
- Take an over-the-counter decongestant pill or a pill such as Mu-cron that contains both a painkiller and a decongestant.
- Use nose drops only for the number of days prescribed. Repeated use of them creates a dependency. Your nasal passages 'forget' how to work on their own and you have to continue using drops to keep nasal passages clear. To avoid picking up germs, never borrow nose drops from others, and don't let anyone else use yours. Throw the drops away after treatment.

SORE THROATS

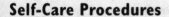

Sore throats range from very slight to pain so severe that even swallowing saliva hurts. Often the cause of all this misery can be either a virus or bacteria. Viral sore throats are the more common of the two and don't respond to antibiotics; bacterial ones do. So it's important to know what kind of infection you have. A sore throat can result from a fungal infection, too. In this case, an antifungal drug is used to treat it.

Bacterial sore throats are most often caused by streptococcus (strep throat) and usually bring a high fever, headaches and swollen, enlarged neck glands with them. Viral sore throats generally don't. But even doctors have trouble diagnosing a sore throat based on symptoms alone. (A child with a bacterial sore throat may have no other symptoms, for example.) In rare cases, an untreated strep throat may lead to serious complications, including abscesses, kidney inflammation or rheumatic heart disease. Because of this risk, your doctor may sometimes take a throat swab. If strep or other bacteria are the culprit, he or she will prescribe an antibiotic. Be sure you take all of the antibiotic.

Questions to Ask

Is it very hard for you to breathe, are you unable to swallow your own saliva, or are you unable to say more than three or four words between breaths? **YES**

NO

Do you have any of the following problems with the sore throat:
• Fever
• Swollen, enlarged neck glands
• Headache
• General achy feeling
• Ear pain
• Bad breath
• Skin rash
• Loss of appetite
• Vomiting
• Abdominal pain
• Chest pain
• Dark urine

YES

NO

Do your tonsils or back of the throat look bright red or have visible pus deposits? **YES**

Does someone else in your family have a strep throat or do you get strep throat often? **YES**

NO

flowchart continued in next column

Has even a mild sore throat lasted more than two weeks? **YES**

NO

Self-Care Procedures

You can take some steps to relieve sore throat discomfort:
• Gargle every few hours with a solution of $1/4$ teaspoon of salt dissolved in $1/2$ a glass of warm water.
• Drink plenty of warm drinks, such as tea (with or without honey) and eat soup.
• Eat and drink cold foods and liquids such as frozen yogurt, ice lollies and ice water.
• Don't smoke. Smoke can aggravate sore throats and make you more susceptible to them.
• Don't eat spicy foods.
• Suck a boiled sweet or a medicated lozenge every so often. (Do not give to children under age five.)
• Take aspirin or paracetamol for the pain or fever (or both). *Note: Do not give aspirin, or any medication containing salicylates, to children under 12 years of age, unless directed by a doctor, due to its association with Reye's syndrome, a potentially fatal condition.*
• Do not get in close contact with anyone you know who has a sore throat.

STYE

A stye is a small boil or bacterial infection in a tiny gland of the eyelid. If the oil-producing glands on the upper or lower rim of the eyelid become infected, they become swollen and painful. A stye is tiny at first, but it can blossom into a bright red, painful sore.

Eventually, a small stye will come to a head and appear yellow, because it accumulates pus. Generally, the tip will face outwards, and the stye will break open and drain on its own.

Questions to Ask

Is it hard for you to see? **YES**

NO

Do you have redness and swelling that hasn't drained within a day or two? **YES**

NO

Do you have a number of styes that appeared at the same time or did you get one after another? **YES**

NO

Self-Care Procedures

You can relieve the discomfort of a stye by following these steps:
- Apply warm (not hot) wet compresses to the affected area three or four times a day for five to 10 minutes at a time.
- Avoid situations that expose your eyes to excessive dust or dirt.
- Don't poke or squeeze the infected area, no matter how tempted you may be to pop the stye. Most styes respond well to home care and don't require further treatment.

TINNITUS (RINGING IN THE EARS)

Imagine hearing a ringing noise in your head that doesn't go away. This maddening noise, called tinnitus, can range in volume from a ring to a roar. Some people are so seriously bothered by it that living a normal life is impossible. In fact, tinnitus can interfere with work, sleep and normal communication with others.

Like a toothache, tinnitus isn't a disease in itself, but a symptom of another problem. Examples are:
- Earwax blocking the ear canals
- Food allergies
- Reactions to medications
- Middle-ear injury or infections
- Blood vessel abnormalities in the brain
- Ear nerve damage (due to exposure to loud noise)
- Anaemia
- Meniere's disease

- Diabetes
- Brain tumours (rarely)

And sometimes, tinnitus is due simply to advancing age. It often accompanies loss of hearing. Occasionally, tinnitus is temporary and will not lead to deafness. Treatment is aimed at finding and treating the problem that causes the tinnitus.

Questions to Ask

Do you have severe pain in the ears, forehead or over the cheekbones, a severe headache, dizziness and/or sudden loss of hearing? **YES**

NO

Have you been taking aspirin or other medications containing salicylates such as Benoral (which is sometimes used to treat arthritis), and do you have these problems with ringing in the ears? **YES**
- Nausea
- Vomiting
- Dizziness
- Rapid breathing
- Hallucinations

NO

flowchart continued in next column

Along with ringing in the ears, do you have one or more of the following?
- Dizziness
- Vertigo
- Unsteadiness in walking
- Loss of balance
- Vomiting
- Difficulty hearing sounds or speech of others

YES

NO

Self-Care Procedures

- For mild cases of tinnitus, play the radio or a 'white noise' tape (white noise is a low, constant sound) in the background to help mask the tinnitus.
- Biofeedback or other relaxation techniques can help you reduce stress, calm down and concentrate, shifting your attention away from the tinnitus.
- Exercise regularly to promote good blood circulation.
- Ask your doctor about a recently developed tinnitus masker, which looks like a hearing aid. Worn on the ear, it makes a subtle noise that masks the tinnitus without interfering with hearing and speech.
- If the noises started during or after travelling in a plane, try pinching your nostrils and blowing through your nose. Chewing gum or sucking a sweet may help prevent the ear popping and

ringing sounds in the ear from happening when you do fly. Also, it is prudent to avoid flying when you have an upper respiratory tract infection.

- Limit your intake of caffeine, alcohol, nicotine and aspirin.
- To prevent damage to the ear, wear earplugs when exposed to loud noises such as heavy machinery.

CHAPTER 2
RESPIRATORY PROBLEMS

ASTHMA

In the UK, asthma affects about one in 10 children and about one in 20 of the total population. The typical symptoms are intermittent wheezing, chest tightness and breathing difficulty. Doctors call asthma an episodic disease because acute attacks alternate with symptom-free periods. Asthma is a physical problem, not an emotional one (although stress, anxiety or frustration can worsen asthma), and it can be severe enough to disrupt people's lives. It is a complex disorder that needs to be treated by a doctor who can monitor its condition.

Asthma cuts down the air flow in the lungs. This makes it hard to breathe and can cause wheezing. (Other things can cause wheezing, too. Something may be stuck in the throat, or there may be an infection. Always tell your doctor about wheezing, especially if your child has it.)

A variety of triggers can set off asthma attacks in susceptible people:
• Having an upper respiratory tract infection or bronchitis
• Breathing an allergen like pollen, mould, animal dander (flakes of dead skin) or particles of dust, smoke or other irritants
• Eating certain foods or taking certain drugs

• Exercising too hard
• Breathing cold air
• Experiencing emotional distress

Asthma attacks range from mild to severe, so treatment varies. Generally, asthma is too complex to treat with over-the-counter preparations. A doctor should monitor your condition.

He or she may prescribe one or more of these for your asthma:
• Bronchodilators, either in oral, inhaled or aerosol form, which open airways to make breathing easier
• Steroids, either in oral or aerosol form, to counteract an allergic reaction, and when other drugs are not sufficient to control your asthma
• Sodium chromoglycate (Intal) to be inhaled before an attack that is triggered by allergies or exercise. This won't work once the attack starts. When used with steroids, though, it may help prevent asthma attacks.

Questions to Ask

Is it so hard for you to breathe that you can't say four or five words between breaths? Or does your chest feel tight? Or do you have wheezing that doesn't go away? **YES**

NO

Does your asthma attack not respond to home treatment or prescribed medicine? **YES**

NO

Do you have signs of an infection (e.g., fever), or are you coughing up anything that is green, yellow or blood-coloured? **YES**

NO

Are your asthma attacks coming more often or getting worse? **YES**

NO

Self-Care Procedures

Asthmatics can do a number of things to help themselves:

- Drink plenty of liquids (2 to 3 litres/3 to 5 pints a day) to keep secretions loose.
- Find out what triggers your asthma, and avoid things that bother you at home and at work.
- Make a special effort to keep your bedroom allergen-free.
  - Sleep with a foam or cotton pillow, not a feather one.
  - Wash mattress covers in hot water every week.
  - Use rugs not carpeting.
  - Don't use curtains.
  - Vacuum and dust often.
- Avoid using perfumes.
- Don't smoke. Try to avoid air pollution.
- Wear a scarf around your mouth and nose when you are outside in cold weather. Doing so will warm the air as you breathe it in and will prevent cold air from reaching sensitive airways.
- Stop exercising if you start to wheeze.
- Don't take foods or medicines that contain sulphites. Sulphites are in wine and many shellfish. They may bother people with asthma.
- Sit up during an asthma attack. Don't lie down.
- Keep your asthma medicine handy. Take it as soon as you start to feel an attack.
- Some people with asthma are allergic to aspirin. Use paracetamol instead.

BRONCHITIS

If you've ever had a cough that felt as though it started down in your feet, or if you've ever started coughing and couldn't stop, you may have had bronchitis.

Bronchitis can be either acute or chronic, depending on how long it lasts and how serious the damage.

Acute bronchitis is generally caused by an infectious agent (like a virus or bacteria) or an environmental pollutant (like tobacco smoke) that attacks the mucus membranes within the windpipe or air passages in your respiratory tract, leaving them red and inflamed. This type often develops in the wake of a sinus infection, cold or other respiratory infection, and can last anywhere from three days to three weeks.

Signs of acute bronchitis are:
- Cough that has little or no sputum
- Chills, low-grade fever (usually less than 38.5°C/101°F)
- Sore throat and muscle aches
- Feeling of pressure behind the breast-bone or a burning feeling in the chest

Treatment may include a doctor's prescription for:
- Bronchodilators (drugs that open up the bronchial passages)
- Antibiotics

In chronic bronchitis, the airways produce too much mucus. It's enough to cause a daily cough that brings up the mucus, continuing for as long as three months or more, for more than two years in a row. Many people, most of them smokers, develop emphysema (destruction of the air sacs) along with chronic bronchitis. Because chronic bronchitis results in abnormal air exchange in the lung and causes permanent damage to the respiratory tract, it's much more serious than acute bronchitis. Signs of chronic bronchitis are:
- A cough that is productive (i.e., one that produces mucus or phlegm)
- Shortness of breath upon exertion (in early stages)
- Shortness of breath at rest (in later stages)

People living in heavily industrialized areas exposed to air pollution, workers exposed to metallic dust or fibres and people who smoke are most susceptible to chronic bronchitis. In fact, cigarette smoking is the most common cause of chronic bronchitis. So stopping smoking is essential and may bring complete relief.

Treatment includes:
- Stopping smoking and avoiding second-hand smoke
- Avoiding or reducing exposure to air pollution and chemical irritants
- Using expectorant cough medicines

Questions to Ask

Is the person who has the cough unable to speak more than four or five words between breaths? Or does the person have purple lips? **YES**

NO

Does the cough occur in a baby and make the baby unable to eat or take a bottle because he or she has difficulty breathing? **YES**

NO

Does the cough occur in an infant younger than three months? **YES**

NO

Does it occur in an infant or young child with rapid breathing and sound like a seal's bark? **YES**

NO

Are any of these problems also present:
- Fever of 38.5°C (101°F) or higher
- Blood in sputum
- Increase in chest pain
- Shortness of breath at rest and when not coughing
- Vomiting

YES

NO

flowchart continued in next column

Have you been exposed to chemicals at work or at home such as those in a new carpet or tobacco smoke? **YES**

NO

Self-Care Procedures

- Take aspirin or paracetamol for fever and aches. *Note: Do not give aspirin, or any medication containing salicylates, to children under 12 years of age, unless directed by a doctor, due to its association with Reye's syndrome, a potentially fatal condition.*
- Rest.
- Drink plenty of liquids such as water, clear soup and tea.
- Don't smoke.
- Stay away from air pollution as much as you can. Stay inside when air pollution is heavy, if you get bronchitis easily.
- Instead of using cough suppressants, use expectorants. Take bronchodilators and/or antibiotics as prescribed by your doctor.

COMMON COLD

As the name suggests, colds are extremely common. Schoolchildren may have as many as 10 a year. Young adults typically have two or three a year although older people may not have any.

The illness usually lasts from three to seven days. Common cold symptoms are:
• Sneezing
• Runny nose
• Fever of 38.5°C (101°F) or less
• Sore throat
• Dry cough

How do you get colds? Colds are caused by viruses. You can get a cold virus from mucus on other people's hands – such as from a handshake – when they have colds. You can also pick up the virus on towels, telephones or money. Then someone else gets the virus from you. It goes on and on. Cold viruses also travel through coughs and sneezes.

Prevention

• Wash your hands often. Keep them away from your nose, eyes and mouth.
• Try not to touch people or their things when they have a cold.
• Get lots of exercise. Eat and sleep well.
• Use a handkerchief or tissues when you sneeze, cough or blow your nose. This helps to keep you from passing your germs to others.

Questions to Ask

Do you have any of these problems with the cold:
• Rapid breathing or trouble breathing
• Wheezing
• Feeling weak or low on energy
• Delirium. (Delirium can make you restless or confused. Sometimes you see things that aren't there. Watch out for this especially in children.)

 YES

NO

Do you have any of these problems with the cold:
• Earache
• Bright red sore throat or sore throat with white spots
• Coughing that lasts more than 10 days
• Coughing up something yellowish-green or grey
• Fever of 38.5°C (191°F) or higher
• A bad smell from the throat, nose or ears

YES

NO

flowchart continued on next page

Do you have pain or swelling over your sinuses that gets worse when you bend over or move your head? (Your sinuses are behind your cheekbones, eyes and forehead.) Watch out for this especially when you also have a fever of 38.5°C (101°F) or higher.

 YES

NO

Self-Care Procedures

Time is the only cure for a cold. Some things can make you feel better, though. Here are some hints for fighting a cold:

• Rest in bed if you have a fever.

• Drink lots of hot or cold drinks. They help clear out your respiratory tract. This can help prevent other problems, like bronchitis.

• Take aspirin, paracetamol or ibuprofen for muscle aches and pains. *Note: Do not give aspirin, or any medication containing salicylates, to children under 12 years of age, unless directed by a doctor, due to its association with Reye's syndrome, a potentially fatal condition.*

• Gargle with warm salt water, drink tea with honey and lemon or suck on throat lozenges for a sore throat. (Do not give lozenges to children under age five.)

• Try steam inhalations.

COUGHS

A lot of things can make you cough:
• An infection
• An allergy
• Cigarette smoke
• Something stuck in your windpipe
• Dry air

Coughing can be a sign of many ailments. Your body uses coughing to clear your lungs and airways. Coughing itself is not the problem. What causes the cough is the problem. There are two kinds of coughs:

Productive – A productive cough brings up mucus or phlegm.

Unproductive – An unproductive cough is dry and doesn't bring up any mucus.

How to treat your cough depends on what kind it is, what caused it and what your other symptoms are. Treat the cause and soothe the irritation. Stay away from smoking and second-hand smoke, especially when you have a cough. Smoke hurts your lungs and makes it harder for your body to fight infection.

Questions to Ask

Do you have these problems:
- Trouble breathing and inability to say more than four or five words between breaths. (A baby or small child may be unable to cry, eat, or drink a bottle.)
- Chest pain
- Fainting
- Coughing up blood

YES

NO

Is the person who has the cough a baby or small child? If so, does he or she have these problems, too:
- The cough sounds like a seal's bark (high and whistling)
- A fever of 39° to 39.5°C (102° to 103°F)

YES

NO

Did the cough start suddenly and last an hour or more without stopping?

YES

NO

Are wheezing, shortness of breath, rapid breathing or swelling of the abdomen, legs and ankles present with the cough?

YES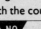

NO

If the person with the cough is an adult, is there a fever of 39°C (102°F) or higher?

YES

NO

Do you have any of these problems with the cough?
- Weight loss for no reason
- Tiredness
- A lot of sweating at night

YES

NO

Does your chest hurt only when you cough, and does the pain go away when you sit up or lean forward?

YES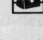

NO

Do you cough up something thick and green-, yellow- or rust-coloured?

YES

NO

Has the cough lasted more than two weeks without getting better?

YES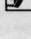

NO

flowchart continued in next column

Self-Care Procedures

For productive coughs (coughs that bring up mucus):
• Drink plenty of liquids. Water helps loosen mucus and soothe a sore throat. Fruit juices are good, too.
• Take a shower or use steam inhalations. The steam can help thin the mucus.
• Ask your pharmacist for an over-the-counter expectorant cough medicine.
• Stop smoking cigarettes, cigars, and/or pipes. Stay away from places where people smoke.

For unproductive coughs (coughs that are dry):
• Drink plenty of liquids.
• Drink hot drinks like tea with lemon and honey to soothe the throat.
• Suck on cough drops or boiled sweets. (Do not give these to children under age five.)
• Take an over-the-counter cough medicine that contains a cough suppressant such as dextromethophan.
• Try a decongestant if you have a runny nose. Nasal secretions dripping down the back of the nose, particularly when lying down can cause a dry cough.
• Make your own cough medicine. Mix one part lemon juice and two parts honey. (Don't give this to children younger than one year.)

Other tips include:

• Don't give children under age five small objects like paper clips and buttons or foods like peanuts and popcorn. A small child can easily get something caught in the throat or windpipe. Even adults should be careful to chew and swallow foods slowly.
• Don't smoke. Stay away from other people's smoke.
• Stay away from chemical gases that can hurt your lungs.
• Exercise. Start gently and work up slowly. You will make your breathing muscles stronger. You will fight infection better, too.

INFLUENZA

'Oh, it's just a touch of flu', some say, as if they had nothing more than a cold. Yet pneumonia and other complications of influenza can be fatal, especially to certain groups of people such as the elderly.

Cold and flu symptoms resemble each other, but they differ in intensity. A cold generally starts out with some minor sniffling and sneezing, flu hits you all at once: You're fine one hour and in bed the next. A cold rarely moves into the lungs; flu can cause pneumonia. You may be able to drag yourself to work with a cold, but with flu you may be too ill to leave your bed.

You probably have flu if you get these symptoms suddenly and severely:
• Dry cough
• Sore throat
• Severe headache
• General muscle aches or backache
• Extreme fatigue
• Chills

- Fever up to 40°C (104°F)
- Pain when you move your eyes, or burning eyes

Muscle aches and fatigue are the main indications of flu. These are normally absent with a cold.

Prevention

To avoid getting flu in the first place:
- Get plenty of rest, eat well, and exercise regularly. These will help you resist picking up flu.
- Get a flu vaccination before each flu season if you are over age 65 or have a chronic medical problem such as diabetes or lung disease that makes it hard for you to fight infection.

Questions to Ask

Do you have any of these problems with your flu:
- Inability to speak more than four or five words between breaths
- Purple lips
- Chest pain
- Coughing up blood
- Fever, stiff neck and lethargy

YES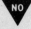

NO

flowchart continued in next column

Do you have any of these problems with the flu:
- Earache
- Sinus pain

YES

NO

Is your fever and/or other symptoms like coughing getting worse?

YES

NO

Have you recently been abroad? Might you have malaria rather than flu?

YES

NO

Have you had flu more than a week and not felt better after trying any of the Self-Care Procedures listed? Or have new symptoms developed?

YES

NO

Have you had any side effects from taking any prescribed or over-the-counter medicine?

YES

NO

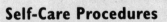

Self-Care Procedures

There's no cure for flu. It has to run its course. Generally, if you are in good health, you can treat the flu on your own. The best way to do this is to get plenty of

rest so your body can fight off the virus.
Try these tips, too:

- Drink lots of hot (but not scalding) drinks. They soothe your throat, help unplug your nose and replace water you lose by sweating.
- Gargle with warm strong tea or warm salt water.
- Use steam inhalations to thin the mucus.
- Suck on cough drops or boiled sweets. (Do not give these to children under age five.)
- Let yourself cough if you are bringing up mucus. Your body needs to get rid of it. Ask your pharmacist for an over-the-counter expectorant cough medicine.
- Don't drink milk or eat dairy foods for a couple of days. They make mucus thick and hard to cough up.
- Wash your hands often. Be sure to wash after blowing your nose and before cooking. This also helps stop you from giving the flu to others.
- Take aspirin, paracetamol or ibuprofen. *Note: Do not give aspirin, or any medication containing salicylates, to children under 12 years of age, unless directed by a doctor, due to its association with Reye's syndrome, a potentially fatal condition.*

CHAPTER 3
SKIN PROBLEMS

ACNE

Acne is a skin condition marked by pimples such as whiteheads, blackheads or even raised, red ones that hurt. These pimples show up on the face, neck, shoulders and/or back. Acne mostly strikes teenagers and young adults. For some, acne or the scars it can leave persist into adulthood. Acne develops when oil ducts below the skin secrete more oil than usual or get clogged with secretions and bacteria. Factors that cause or worsen acne include:

- Normal increase in the levels of the hormone androgen during adolescence
- Changes in hormone levels before a woman's menstrual period or during pregnancy
- Rich moisturizing lotions or heavy or greasy make-up
- Emotional stress
- Rarely, cooking oils, tar or creosote in the air. Creosote is sometimes used as a wood preservative.
- Birth control pills, steroids, anti-epilepsy medications and lithium (the latter used to treat some forms of depression)

Most cases of acne can be treated with the Self-Care Procedures listed. If these are not enough, ask your doctor about the various alternatives available on prescription.

Questions to Ask

Is your acne very bad and do you have signs of an infection with it (e.g., fever and swelling)? **YES**

NO

Are the pimples big and painful? **YES**

NO

Have you tried the Self-Care Procedures and they haven't helped, or have the Self-Care Procedures made your skin worse? **YES**

NO

Self-Care Procedures

Time is the only cure for acne, but these tips may help:

- Keep your skin clean. Wash often with plain soap and water. Use a facecloth. Work the soap into your skin gently for a minute or two. Rinse well.
- Use a clean facecloth every day. Bacteria, which can give you more pimples, love a wet facecloth.

- Try an astringent lotion, de-greasing pads or a face scrub.
- Leave your skin alone! Don't squeeze, scratch or poke at pimples. They can get infected and leave scars.
- Use an over-the-counter lotion or cream that contains benzoyl peroxide. Ask your pharmacist for advice. (Some people are allergic to benzoyl peroxide. Try a little on your arm first to make sure it doesn't hurt your skin.) Follow the directions.
- Wash after you exercise or sweat.
- Wash your hair at least twice a week.
- For men: Wrap a warm towel around your face before you shave. This will make your beard softer. Always shave in the direction the hair grows.
- Sunlight may help but don't overdo it. Avoid the sun completely if you are taking a prescription medicine that causes a bad reaction in combination with sunlight (your doctor will advise you on this).
- Use only water-based make-up. Don't use greasy or oily creams, lotion or make-up.

ATHLETE'S FOOT

It's itchy. It's persistent. It's contagious. It smells bad. And it attacks the skin between the toes (usually the third and fourth). What is it? A fungal infection of the skin, better known as athlete's foot.

People usually get athlete's foot from walking barefoot over wet floors around swimming pools, locker rooms and public showers that are contaminated with the fungus, which feasts on moisture. Athlete's foot has these signs and symptoms:
- Moist, soft red or grey-white scales on the feet, especially between the toes
- Cracked, peeling, dead skin areas
- Itching
- Sometimes small blisters on the feet

Questions to Ask

Do you have signs of athlete's foot and are you diabetic or do you have poor leg circulation? YES

NO

Do you have a fever and/or is the infection spreading or getting worse despite doing the Self-Care Procedures listed? YES

NO

Self-Care Procedures

If you get athlete's foot:
- Wash your feet twice a day, especially between your toes, and dry the area thoroughly.
- Apply an over-the-counter antifungal powder, cream or spray between your toes and inside your socks and shoes.
- Wear clean socks made of cotton or wool. (Natural fibres absorb moisture.)

Change your socks during the day to help your feet stay dry.
- Wear shoes made of leather rather than plastic. Also, try to wear shoes such as sandals that provide some ventilation.
- Don't wear the same shoes every day. Alternate pairs and let each pair air out between wearings.

BURNS

Burns can result from dry heat (fire), moist heat (steam, hot liquids), electricity, chemicals, or radiation (including sunlight). Treatment for burns depends on:
- The depth of the burn (whether it is first-, second- or third-degree)
- How much area of the body is affected
- The location of the burn

First-degree burns affect only the outer layer of skin. The skin area appears dry, red and mildly swollen. Such burns are painful and sensitive to the touch. Mild sunburn and brief contact with a heat source (e.g., a hot iron) are examples of this type of burn. First-degree burns should feel better within a day or two. They should heal in about a week if there are no complications. (See Self-Care Procedures.)

Second-degree burns affect the lower layers of the skin as well as the outer skin. They are painful and swollen, and show redness and blisters. The skin also develops a weepy, watery surface. Examples of second-degree burns are severe sunburn and burns caused by hot liquids. Self-Care Procedures can be used to treat many second-degree burns, depending on where the burns are and the size of the affected area.

Third-degree burns affect the outer and deeper skin layers as well as any underlying tissue and organs. They appear black and white and charred. The skin is swollen and underlying tissue is often exposed. The pain felt with third-degree burns may be less than with first- or second-degree burns or none at all because nerve endings may be destroyed. Pain may be felt around the margin of the affected area, however. Third-degree burns usually result from electric shocks, burning clothes, severe petrol fires, etc. They always require emergency treatment. They may result in hospitalization and sometimes require skin grafts.

Questions to Ask

Is the burn a third-degree burn? (Is there absence of pain, the presence of charred, black and white skin, and exposure of tissue under the skin?) **YES**

NO

flowchart continued on next page

Is the burn a second-degree burn (affecting more than the outer skin and with signs of blistering over an area more than 2–3 cm/1 in in diameter) on the face, hands, feet, genitals or on any joint (elbow, knee, shoulder, etc.)?

YES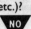

NO

Is the burn a second-degree burn (affecting more than the outer skin and with signs of blistering over an area more than 2–3 cm/1 in in diameter) somewhere other than the face, hands, feet, genitals or a joint?

YES

NO

Was the burn caused by an electrical contact?

YES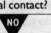

NO

Is the burn victim an infant or a young child?

YES

NO

Self-Care Procedures

For first-degree burns:

- Cool the area right away. Place the affected area in a container of cold water or under cold running water. Do this for at least 10 minutes or until the pain is relieved. This will also reduce the amount of skin damage.
- Do not apply ice or cold water for too long a time. This may result in complete numbness leading to frostbite.
- Keep the area uncovered and elevated, if possible. Apply a dry dressing if necessary.
- Do not use butter or other ointments.
- Avoid using local anaesthetic sprays and creams. They can slow healing and may lead to allergic reactions in some people.
- Call your doctor if after two days you show signs of infection (fever of 38.5°C/101°F or higher, chills, and increased redness, swelling or pus in the infected area) or if the affected area is still painful.
- Take aspirin, paracetamol or ibuprofen to relieve pain. *Note: Do not give aspirin, or any medication containing salicylates, to children under 12 years of age, unless directed by a doctor, due to its association with Reye's syndrome, a potentially fatal condition.*

For second-degree burns (that are not extensive and are less than 7.5 cm/3 in in diameter):
- Immerse the affected area in cold (not ice) water for at least 10 minutes or until the pain subsides.

- Dip clean cloths in cold water, wring them out and apply them over and over again to the burned area for as long as an hour. Blot the area dry. Do not rub.
- Do not break any blisters that have formed.
- Avoid applying antiseptic sprays, ointments, creams. Once dried, dress the area with a single layer of loose gauze that does not stick to the skin. Hold gauze in place with adhesive tape positioned well away from the burned area.
- Change the dressing the next day and every two days after that.
- Prop the burn area higher than the rest of the body, if possible.
- Call your doctor if there are signs of infection (e.g., fever of 38.5°C/101°F or higher, chills, and increased redness and swelling or pus in the affected area) or if the burn shows no sign of improvement after two days.

COLD HANDS AND FEET

Some people wear mittens and heavy socks all the year round, indoors and out, because their hands and feet always feel cold. Factors that may make the extremities feel cold include:
- Poor circulation due to coronary heart disease
- Raynaud's disease (disorder that affects the flow of blood to the fingers and sometimes to the toes)
- Frostbite
- Working with vibrating equipment (like a pneumatic drill)

- A side effect of taking certain medications
- An underlying disease affecting blood flow in the tiny blood vessels of the skin. (Women smokers may be prone to this condition.)
- Stress

Symptoms to look for are:
- Fingers or toes turning pale white or blue, then red, in response to cold
- Tingling or numbness
- Pain during the white phase of discoloration

Questions to Ask

Have your hands or feet had prolonged exposure to below-freezing temperatures which may have resulted in frostbite? (Frostbite symptoms are tingling and redness followed by paleness [white or blueish appearance] and numbness of affected areas.) **YES**

 NO

Do your hands or feet turn pale, then blue then red, and get painful and numb when exposed to the cold or stress? **YES**

 NO

Self-Care Procedures

If wearing gloves and wool socks and staying indoors where it's warm are nuisances and don't help, try these tips:
- Don't smoke. It impairs circulation.
- Avoid caffeine. It constricts blood vessels.
- Avoid handling cold objects. Use ice tongs to pick up ice cubes, for instance.
- With fingers outstretched, swing your arms in large circles, like the sails of a windmill. This may increase blood flow to the fingers. (Do not follow this tip if you have back problems.)
- Do not wear footwear that is tight-fitting.
- Wiggle your toes. It may help keep them warm by increasing blood flow.
- Make sure to keep your whole body warm not just your hands and feet. A warm body sends more blood out to the extremities.

CORNS AND CALLOUSES

All too often, corns and callouses are the price we pay for neglecting our feet. Corns and callouses are very much alike; they just differ in where they occur.

Corns show up on the bony area on top of the toes and the skin between the toes. Corns feel hard to the touch, are tender and have a roundish appearance. A small, clear spot may form in the centre.

Callouses can occur on any part of the body that goes through repeated pressure or irritation. Common places are on the heels or balls of the feet, on the hands and on the knees. Callouses are flat, painless thickenings of the skin.

Corns and callouses form as a protective response. They are extra cells made in a skin area that gets repeated rubbing or squeezing from such things as:
- Footwear that fits poorly
- Activities that put pressure on the hands, knees and feet

If Self-Care Procedures do not get rid of corns and callouses, a family doctor or chiropodist may need to be consulted. He or she can scrape away the hardened tissue and peel away the corn with stronger solutions.

Questions to Ask

Do you have any signs of infection (fever, or swelling, redness, pus sacs or puffiness near the corn)? **YES**

NO

Do you have circulation problems or diabetes mellitus? **YES**

NO

Do you have one or both of these problems even after following the Self-Care Procedures:
- Continued or worse pain
- No improvement after two to three weeks

YES

NO

Self-Care Procedures

For corns: Never pick at corns or use nail scissors or clippers, a razor blade or any other sharp tool to cut off corns. You may injure your skin or trigger an infection. Instead:

• Get rid of shoes that fit badly, especially if they squeeze your toes together.
• Soak your feet in warm water to soften the corn.
• Cover the corn with a protective, non-medicated pad, usually available in chemists. (A piece of foam rubber or moleskin will do at a pinch.)
• If the out layers of a corn have peeled away, ask your pharmacist for an over-the-counter corn liquid containing salicylic acid. Apply the liquid as directed and cover the area with a plaster.

For callouses: Never try to get rid of a callous by cutting it with a sharp tool. Instead:

• Soak your feet in warm water to soften the callous, then pat dry.
• Rub the callous gently with a pumice stone.
• Cover callouses with protective pads, available in chemists.
• Check for poorly fitting shoes or other sources of pressure that may lead to callouses.
• Wear gloves if doing a hobby or work that puts pressure on the hands.
• Wear knee pads for activities that put pressure on your knees.

CUTS, SCRAPES AND PUNCTURES

Cuts, scrapes and punctures all make you bleed, but there are differences between them:

• Cuts slice the skin open. Cover cuts so they won't get infected.
• Scrapes hurt only the top part of your skin. They can hurt more than cuts, but they heal quicker.
• Puncture wounds stab deep. Leave punctures open so they won't get infected.

You can treat most cuts, scrapes and puncture wounds yourself. But you should go to a hospital Accident and Emergency Department if you are bleeding a lot, or if you are hurt very badly.

Blood gets thicker after bleeding for a few minutes due to clotting, which slows down bleeding. Press on the cut to help slow down the bleeding. You may have to apply firm pressure for 10 minutes for a bad cut. Don't keep looking to see if the bleeding has stopped. Sometimes a cut needs stitches. Stitches help the cut heal.

Questions to Ask

Is the bleeding from a cut, scrape or puncture wound severe:
- Is the person in shock?
- Does blood spurt from the wound?
- Has the person lost a lot of blood? (12 ml/¼ pt for an adult, less for a child)?
- Is the cut still bleeding a lot after 10 minutes of applied pressure?

YES

NO

Does the cut need stitches?
- Is it deep? (Does it go down to the muscle or bone?)
- Is it on the head or face?
- Is it longer than 2.5 cm (1 in) on a body part that bends such as an elbow, knee or finger?
- Do the edges of the cut skin hang open?

YES

NO

Is the cut still bleeding after 20 minutes of applied pressure, even if it is a small cut?

YES

NO

flowchart continued in next column

Are there signs of infection a day or two after the injury:
- Fever of 38.5°C (101°F) or higher
- Redness, swelling, tenderness at or around the wound
- Pain that gets worse instead of better

YES

NO

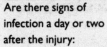

Self-Care Procedures

For cuts and scrapes:
- Clean around the wound with soap and water. (It doesn't matter if some gets into the cut, but it may hurt.)
- Press on the cut to stop the bleeding. Do this up for up to 10 minutes if you need to. Use a sterile bandage or a clean cloth. Use a clean hand if you don't have a bandage or cloth. (Dry gauze can stick to the wound, so try not to use it.) Don't use a sticking plaster.
- Press on the cut again if it keeps bleeding. Get help if it is still bleeding after 20 or more minutes. Keep pressing on it while you wait for help.
- Lift the part of the body with the cut higher than the person's heart. This slows down blood flow to that spot.
- Put antiseptic cream on the cut when it is clean and dry. Use a sterile cloth or cotton swab.

- Put one or more sticking plasters on the cut. Do it this way:

Put the sticking plaster across the cut so it can help hold the cut together.
- The sides of the cut should touch, but only just. Don't let them overlap.
- Don't touch the cut with your hand.
- Use more than one sticking plaster or use gauze held with adhesive tape for a long cut.
- For scrapes, use gauze held with adhesive tape.
- Leave the bandage on for 24 hours. Change the bandage every day or two. Change it more often if you need to. Be careful when you take the bandage off. You don't want to make the cut bleed again. Wet the gauze before you pull it off.
- Take paracetamol or ibuprofen for pain. Don't take aspirin unless your doctor tells you to. Aspirin can keep blood from clotting if you take it for a long time.
- Call your doctor right away or go to the nearest hospital Accident and Emergency Department if you have not had a tetanus booster in the last 10 years. Ask if you need a booster.

For puncture wounds that cause minor bleeding:
- Let the wound bleed to clean itself out.
- Take out anything that caused the puncture. Use clean tweezers. *Don't pull anything out of a puncture wound if blood gushes from it or if it has been bleeding a lot. Seek emergency treatment.*
- Wash the wound with warm water and soap, or take a bath or shower to clean it.

- Leave the wound open. You can cover it with a bandage if it is big or still bleeds a little.

ECZEMA

Eczema is a chronic skin problem. A chronic problem lasts a long time and can come and go. Most people get eczema on the head, face, neck or the insides of their elbows, wrists and knees. It looks like small blisters and crusty scales. Both children and adults get eczema. It runs in families. People who have asthma often have eczema, too. Eczema is usually worse when you are a child. Then it gets better and may even go away. But some people have eczema all their lives. The following can worsen eczema in some people:
- Woollen clothes
- Sweating
- Stress
- Weather conditions, especially very hot, humid weather
- Foods like eggs, milk, seafood and wheat
- Cosmetics, dyes, medicines, deodorants, skin lotions and other things that may cause allergy

Questions to Ask

Are there any signs of infection with the eczema? Do you have a fever? Or is the eczema very crusty and runny?

YES →

NO ↓

Has the rash lasted for a long time?

YES →

NO ↓

Self-Care Procedures

Your doctor should treat eczema. But you can do a lot to make it better:
- Don't take baths too often. Add bath oil to the water. Or take quick showers.
- Use warm water instead of hot when you take a bath or shower.
- Don't use soap on the eczema.
- Avoid woollen clothes and blankets.
- Use a light, non-greasy lotion on your skin after you wash. Pick one that's unscented and lanolin free.
- Try to avoid sweating. For example, don't wear too many clothes for the weather.
- Wear rubber gloves when you do housework. Try latex gloves lined with cotton.
- Stay away from food, chemicals, cosmetics and other things that make your eczema worse.
- Try not to scratch! Scratching eczema only makes it worse. It can get infected. Keep your fingernails short.

FROSTBITE

The effects of frostbite are extremely painful. Yet preventing frostbite is remarkably simple.

Frostbite looks like a serious heat burn, but it's actually body tissue that's frozen and, in severe cases, dead. Most often, frostbite affects the toes, fingers, earlobes, chin and tip of the nose (i.e., unprotected extremities that freeze quickly). Danger signs are pain (initially), swelling, white skin, then numbness and eventually loss of function and absence of pain. Blisters may also develop.

Sheer cold causes frostbite, but wind chill speeds up heat loss and increases the risk. Depending on how long you're exposed and how cold or windy it is, frostbite can set in very slowly, or very quickly, before you know what's happening.

Prevention

Needless to say, frostbite is something you should try to prevent. Here are some 'keep warm' precautions to take if you expect to spend any length of time in the cold:
- Wear layers of clothing. Many layers of thin clothing are warmer than one bulky layer. The air spaces trap body warmth close to the skin, insulating the body against cold. For example, wear two or three pairs of light- or standard-weight socks instead of one heavy pair.
- Avoid drinking alcohol or smoking cigarettes. Alcohol causes blood to lose

heat rapidly, and smoking slows down blood circulation to the extremities.

- Try to avoid being out of doors in extremely low temperatures and high winds.

- Never massage a frostbitten area.
- Protect exposed area from the cold. It is more sensitive to further injury.

Questions to Ask

After exposure to cold temperature, do you experience:
- Pain, swelling, tingling or burning of the skin
- Skin colour changing from white to red to purple
- Blisters
- Shivering
- Slurred speech
- Memory loss

Self-Care Procedures

The old advice that says you should treat frostbite by rubbing the area with snow or soaking it in cold water is wrong. This treatment is ineffective and dangerous. Instead:

- Warm the affected area by soaking in a bath of warm water (38.5° to 40°C/101° to 104°F).
- Stop when the affected area becomes red, not when sensation returns.
- Keep exposed area elevated.

HAIR LOSS

Most men and women experience hair loss as they get older; indeed, most men have some degree of baldness by the age of 60. This is quite normal and affects some persons more than others, especially if baldness runs in the family. Sudden or abnormal hair loss could, however, result from:

- Taking certain medications (like some used in treating cancer, circulatory disorders, ulcers or arthritis)
- Following a crash diet
- Hormonal changes (such as at the menopause)
- A prolonged or serious illness
- Temporarily after having a baby

Some medical conditions lead to hair loss. These need treatment. They include:
- Hypothyroidism (underactive thyroid gland)
- Ringworm (a fungal infection that affects the scalp and/or hairs themselves)
- Alopecia areata, which causes areas of patchy hair loss, but does not affect the scalp. This condition may improve with treatment, but can also disappear within 18 months without treatment. Doctors may prescribe a topical steroid to be used once or twice a day.

For cosmetic reasons, some people wear wigs or toupees. Surgical hair transplant operations are a treatment option for both men and women, in very select cases. (Wear a hat or use a sunscreen with a sun protection factor [SPF] of 15 or more on the bald parts of your head when your head is exposed to the sun. The risk of sunburn and skin cancer on the scalp increases with baldness.)

Questions to Ask

Do you experience one or more of the following:
• Unexplained fatigue and weight gain
• Feeling the cold
• Numbness and tingling of hands and feet
• Coarse skin and hair
• Deepened or hoarse voice
• Depression
• Decreased sex drive

YES

NO

Has the hair loss occurred suddenly and in patches on the head? Is the scalp affected in any way, such as with red or grey-green scales?

YES

NO

Are there signs of infection (e.g., redness, tenderness, swelling and/or pain) at the site of hair loss?

YES

NO

flowchart continued in next column

Does the hair loss occur from uncontrollably pulling out patches of hair?

YES

NO

Have you begun losing your hair only after taking prescribed medicine for high blood pressure, high cholesterol, ulcers or arthritis?

YES

NO

Do you want to find out about hair implants to treat naturally occurring hair thinning or baldness?

YES

NO

Self-Care Procedures

To protect your hair from damage and loss:
• Avoid damaging hair care practices or use them infrequently. These include: plaiting, use of rollers; bleaching, dyeing, perming, straightening; use of heated rollers and tongs, and hair dryers, especially on a high setting.
• Use gentle shampoos and conditioners
• Leave your hair to dry naturally or pat it dry with a towel
• If your hair is damaged, cut it short or change your hairstyle to one that requires less damaging hair care practices.

- Take measures (e.g., yoga and other relaxation techniques) to reduce anxiety if this results in pulling out patches of hair.
- Don't be taken in by fraudulent claims for vitamin formulas, massage oils, lotions or ointments that promise to cure baldness.
- Ask your doctor for a substitute medication if you are taking one that has caused hair loss. (Obviously, this may not be feasible with anticancer drugs.)

- Infections
- Inhalants (especially pollen, mould spores or airborne chemicals)
- Insect bites
- Rubbing or putting pressure on the skin
- Exposure to chemicals
- Malignant or connective tissue disease

The cause of hives is not always known. But if you can identify the triggers (try keeping a diary), you may be able to prevent future outbreaks.

HIVES

Hives, also called nettle rash or urticaria, are red, raised, itchy weals. They appear, sometimes in clusters, on the face, trunk of the body, and, less often, on the scalp, hands or feet. Like the Cheshire cat in *Alice's Adventures in Wonderland*, hives can change shape, fade, then rapidly reappear. A single hive lasts less than 24 hours, but after an attack new ones may crop up for up to six weeks. About one in five people are estimated to suffer from hives at some time in their lives.

Hives can be (but aren't always) an allergic response to something you touched, inhaled or swallowed. Some common causes of hives include:
- Reactions to medications such as aspirin and penicillin
- Animal dander (flakes of dead skin)
- Cold temperatures
- Emotional or physical stress (including exercise)
- Foods (especially chocolate, nuts, shellfish or tomatoes)

Questions to Ask

Do you have any of these problems:
- Shortness of breath and breathing difficulties
- Wheezing, dizziness
- Swollen lips tongue, and/or throat

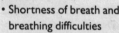

YES

NO

Did hives start after recently taking a medication?

 YES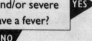

NO

Do you have itching that is constant and/or severe or do you have a fever?

YES

NO

Self-Care Procedures

Here are some tips for treating a mild case of hives:
- Don't take hot baths or showers. Heat worsens most rashes and makes them itch more.
- Apply cold compresses or take a warm bath.
- Wear loose-fitting clothing.
- Relax as much as possible. Studies have shown that relaxation therapy and even hypnosis help ease the itching and discomfort of hives.
- Ask your doctor whether or not you should take an antihistamine and ask him or her to recommend one. Antihistamines can help relieve itching and suppress hives. (Keep in mind that some antihistamines can cause drowsiness and may make it dangerous for you to drive or perform other tasks requiring alertness.)
- Avoid taking aspirin or ibuprofen. They may aggravate hives.

INSECT STINGS

Warm-weather months often include run-ins with bees, wasps, mosquitos, fleas, spiders, etc.

As you'd expect, most people who have been stung know it. The most common symptoms are limited areas of pain and swelling with redness and itching. Beyond that, the symptoms of bee and wasp stings vary, depending on where you're stung and how sensitive you are to the sting.

People who are allergic to insect stings may have a severe reaction known as anaphylactic shock (even if they've never had an allergic reaction to a sting before). The symptoms of a severe anaphylactic reaction include generalized swelling, wheezing, difficult breathing, a severe drop in blood pressure and sometimes coma and death. Needless to day, this is a medical emergency, so if you start to have a serious reaction to a sting, get medical help immediately.

If you've ever experienced an allergic reaction to an insect sting in the past, you should carry an emergency medical kit containing adrenaline (a drug to stop the body-wide reaction) and a hypodermic needle to inject it, an antihistamine, and a Medic Alert bracelet that lets others know you're allergic to insect stings. Also, people who have had severe reactions to bee or wasp stings should consider desensitizing injections as a protective measure.

Prevention

How can you avoid getting stung?
- Keep foods and drinks tightly covered. (Bees love sweet foods and soft drinks.)
- Avoid sweet-smelling colognes. Wear an insect repellent instead.
- Avoid looking like a flower. Choose white or neutral colours that won't attract bees.
- Wear snug clothing that covers your arms and legs, and don't go barefoot.
- Treat animals for fleas.

Questions to Ask

If you are stung by an insect, do you have these problems:
- Generalized swelling
- Throat feels closed up
- Wheezing
- Difficulty in breathing and/or swallowing
- Slurred speech
- Confusion
- Hives all over the body

YES

NO

Were you stung in the mouth or on the tongue?

YES

NO

Has the bitten area become increasingly red, swollen, warm and tender?

YES

NO

Have the symptoms not been relieved by the Self-Care Procedures listed?

YES

NO

Self-Care Procedures

- Gently scrape out the sting, if there is one, as soon as possible.
- Don't pull or squeeze the sting. It contains venom, and you'll end up re-stinging yourself. (This applies to bees only; wasps and hornets don't lose their sting.)
- Clean the stung area with soapy water.
- Apply ice to the stung area immediately; it will minimize discomfort and prevent swelling and itching.
- Take aspirin or paracetamol or ibuprofen for the pain, and/or an antihistamine for the itching and swelling (provided you don't have to avoid these drugs for medical reasons). *Note: Do not give aspirin, or any medication containing salicylates, to children under 12 years of age, unless directed by a doctor, due to its association with Reye's syndrome, a potentially fatal condition.*

SHINGLES

Shingles (herpes zoster) is a skin disorder triggered by the chicken pox virus (varicella zoster) that many people first encounter as a child.

This virus is thought to lie dormant in the spinal cord until later in life. Shingles most often occur between the ages of 50 and 70 in both men and women. Even though shingles is not as contagious as chicken pox, infants and people whose immunity is low should not be exposed to it. Besides ageing, the risks for getting shingles increase with:
- Hodgkin's disease or other cancer
- Any illness in which infection-fighting systems are below par
- The use of anticancer drugs or any drugs that suppress the immune system (e.g., corticosteroids)

- Stress or trauma, either emotional or physical

Symptoms of shingles include:
- Pain, itching or tingling sensation before the rash appears.
- A rash of painful red blisters, which later crust over. Most often, the rash appears on the trunk or side of the face, and sometimes affects the eye. Only one side of the face or body is usually affected. Shingles is rarely present on both sides of the body.
- Though rare, fever and general weakness sometimes occur.

After the crusts fall off (usually within three weeks), pain can persist in the area of the rash. This usually goes away on its own after one to six months. Chronic pain can, however, last for months or years. The older you are, the greater the chances are that this is the case and the recovery time may also take longer.

Most cases of shingles are mild but some can result in chronic, severe pain. So, to be on the safe side, if you get shingles let your doctor know.

Treatment for shingles includes:
- Pain relief with analgesics (codeine may sometimes be prescribed)
- Prescription medicines: antiviral drugs such as acyclovir or famciclovir, usually in tablet form. The sooner these medicines are started, the better the results.
- An antibiotic if the blisters become infected

Questions to Ask

With shingles, are you over 60 years of age, taking anticancer or other immunosuppressive drugs or have a chronic illness? **YES**

NO

Has the shingles affected your eyes? **YES**

NO

Do the blisters itch uncontrollably or are they very painful? **YES**

NO

Do you have a fever and/or general weakness? **YES**

NO

Do any symptoms of shingles make you uncomfortable? **YES**

NO

Self-Care Procedures

Following are things you can do (along with your doctor's recommendations) to help relieve an active outbreak of shingles:
- Take an over-the-counter pain reliever such as paracetamol, aspirin or ibuprofen, unless your doctor has given

you a prescription painkiller. Ask your doctor which over-the-counter painkiller is best for you. *Note: Do not give aspirin, or any medication containing salicylates, to children under 12 years of age, unless directed by a doctor, due to its association with Reye's syndrome, a potentially fatal condition.*

- If possible, keep sores open to the air. Don't bandage them unless you live with or are around children or adults who have not yet had chicken pox. They could pick up chicken pox from exposure to shingles.
- Don't wear restrictive clothing that irritates the area of the body where sores are present.
- Wash blisters, but never scrub them.
- Apply cool compresses, calamine lotion or baking soda to help alleviate the symptoms.

SKIN RASHES

Skin rashes come in all forms and sizes. Some are raised bumps, others are flat red blotches. Some are itchy blisters; others are patches of rough skin. Most rashes are harmless and clear up on their own within a few days. A few may need medical attention. The skin is one of the first areas of the body to react when exposed to something you or your child is allergic to.

The chart on page 51 lists information on some common skin rashes.

Questions to Ask

Are you having trouble breathing or swallowing, or is the tongue swollen? **YES**

 NO

Do you have any of the following:
- Fever
- Headache
- Sore throat
- A fine red rash that feels rough like sandpaper
- Joint pain along with a rash

YES

 NO

Are there any large, fluid-filled blisters present or pus or swelling around the spots? **YES**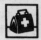

 NO

Have you recently been exposed to someone with a severe sore throat? **YES**

 NO

If your child has nappy rash, are there also blisters or small red patches that appear outside the nappy area, for example on the chest? **YES**

 NO

flowchart continued on next page

When the rash started, were you taking any medications or were you stung by an insect?

YES

 NO

Is the rash getting worse, keeping you from sleeping and/or do the Self-Care Procedures not relieve symptoms?

YES

 NO

Self-Care Procedures

Heat rash is best treated by staying in a cool, dry area. It will usually disappear within two to three days if you keep the skin cool. Things you can do:
- Take a bath in cool water, without soap, every couple of hours.
- Let your skin dry without using a towel.
- Apply calamine lotion to very itchy spots.
- Don't use ointments and creams that can block the sweat gland pores.
  To treat nappy rash in a child:
- Change nappies as soon as they become wet or soiled (even at night if the rash is extensive).
- Wash your baby with plenty of warm water (don't use disposable wipes) to prevent irritating the skin. If the skin appears irritated, apply a light coat of a barrier cream after the skin is completely dry. Ask your health visitor for advice.

- Keep the skin dry and exposed to air.
- Before putting on a fresh nappy, keep your baby's bottom naked on a soft, fluffy towel for 10 to 15 minutes.
- Put nappies on loosely so air can circulate under them. Avoid ones with tight leg bands.
- Don't use plastic pants until the rash is gone.
- Wash cloth nappies in mild soap. Add 1/2 cup of vinegar to your rinse water to help remove what's left of the soap.

Hives can be eased if you:
- Take an antihistamine (ask your pharmacist for advice). Note that some antihistamines cause drowsiness.
- Cool off. Rub an ice cube over the hives, drape a facecloth dipped in cool water over the affected areas or take a cool-water bath.
- Rub your body with calamine lotion, witch hazel or zinc oxide.
- Find and eliminate the cause of the allergic reaction if possible.

For cradle cap in babies:
- Use an anti-dandruff shampoo once a day, massaging your baby's scalp with a soft brush or facecloth for five minutes.
- Soften the hard crusts by applying olive oil on the scalp before washing your child's hair. Be sure to thoroughly wash the oil out completely. Otherwise, the cradle cap condition may worsen.

To protect yourself from Lyme disease (a tick-borne infection):
- Wear long pants tucked into socks and long-sleeve shirts when you walk

through fields and forests. Light-coloured, tightly woven clothing is best.
- Inspect yourself for ticks after outdoor activities.
Remove any ticks found on the skin as follows:
  - Use tweezers to grasp the tick as close to the skin as possible.
  - Pull in a steady upward motion.
  - Try not to crush the tick because the secretions released may spread disease.
  - Wash the wound area and your hands with soap and water after removing ticks.
  - Save any removed ticks in a jar and take them to the doctor to aid in the diagnosis of Lyme disease.

To treat chicken pox:

The goals in treating chicken pox are to reduce and relieve the itching for comfort and to prevent scratching off of the scabs which could start a secondary infection and/or leave scars.

For chicken pox in children:
- Encourage your child not to scratch the scabs. Keep him or her busy with other activities.
- Give your child a cool bath without soap, every three to four hours for the first couple of days for 15 to 20 minutes at a time. Add $1/2$ cup of bicarbonate of soda to the bath water. Pat, do not rub, your child dry. Or dip a facecloth in cool water and place it on the itchy areas.
- Apply calamine lotion to the spots for temporary relief.
- Trim your child's fingernails to prevent infection caused by opened blisters.

Scratching off the crusty scabs may leave permanent scars.
- Cover the hands of infants with cotton socks if they are scratching their sores.
- Wash your child's hands three times a day with an antibacterial soap to avoid infecting the open blisters.
- Keep your child cool and calm. Heat and sweating make the itching worse. Also, keep your child out of the sun. Further spots will occur on parts of the skin that are exposed to the sun.
- Give your child an over-the-counter antihistamine if the itching is severe or stops your child from sleeping. (Ask your pharmacist for advice and see the label for proper dosage.)
- Give your child paracetamol suspension for the fever. *Note: Do not give aspirin, or any medication containing salicylates, to children under 12 years of age, unless directed by a doctor, due to its association with Reye's syndrome, a potentially fatal condition.*
- Give your child soft foods and cold fluids if he or she has sores in the mouth. Do not offer salty foods or citrus fruits that may irritate the sores.
- Reassure your child that the spots are not serious and will go away in a week or so.

For eczema, see Self-Care Procedures listed on page 41.

COMMON SKIN RASHES

CONDITION OR ILLNESS	CAUSES	WHAT RASH LOOKS LIKE	SKIN AREAS AFFECTED	OTHER SYMPTOMS
Nappy Rash	Dampness and the interaction of urine and the skin	Small patches of rough skin, tiny pimples or raw areas	Buttocks, thighs, genitals	Soreness, no itching
Cradle Cap	Hormones that pass through the placenta before birth	Scaly, crusty rash (in babies under 1 year)	Starts behind the ears and spreads to the scalp	Fine, oily scales
Heat Rash (Prickly Heat)	Blocked off sweat glands	Small red pimples, pink blotchy skin	Chest, waist, back, armpits, groin	Itching (may be a result of fever)
'Roseola	Herpes virus type–6	Flat, rosy red rash	Chest, abdomen	High fever 2 to 4 days before rash – child feels only mildly ill during fever
'Fifth Disease; Slapcheek Disease	Human parvovirus B19	Red rash of varying shades that fades to a flat, lacy pattern (rash comes and goes)	Red rash on facial cheeks, lacy rash can also appear on arms and legs	Mild disease with no other symptoms or a slight runny nose and sore throat
Eczema	Allergens	Dry, red, cracked skin, blisters that ooze and crust over, sufficient scratching leads to a thickened rough skin	On cheeks in infants, on neck, wrists, inside elbows and backs of knees in older children	Moderate to intense itching (may only itch first, then rash appears hours to days later)
'·²Chicken Pox	Varicella/herpes zoster virus	Flat red spots that become raised resembling small pimples. These develop into small blisters that break and crust over	Back, chest and abdomen first, then rest of body	Fatigue and mild fever 24 hours before rash appears – intense itching
'Scarlet Fever	Bacterial infection (streptococcal)	Rough, bright red rash (feels like sandpaper)	Face, neck, elbows, armpits, groin (spreads rapidly to entire body)	High fever, weakness before rash, sore throat, peeling of the skin afterwards (especially palms)

CONDITION OR ILLNESS	CAUSES	WHAT RASH LOOKS LIKE	SKIN AREAS AFFECTED	OTHER SYMPTOMS
'Impetigo	Bacterial infection of the skin	In infants, pus-filled blisters and red skin. In older children, golden crusts on red sores	Arms, legs, face and around nose first, then most of body	Sometimes fever – occasional itching
Hives	Allergic reaction to food, insect bites, viral infection, drug or other substance	Raised red bumps with pale centres (resemble mosquito bites), shape, size and location of spots can change rapidly	Any area	Itching – in extreme cases, swelling of throat, difficulty breathing (may need emergency care)
Lyme Disease	Bacterial infection spread by deer tick bite(s)	Red rash that looks like a bull's-eye: raised edges surround the tick bites with pale centres in the middle. Rash starts to fade after a couple of days	Exposed skin areas where ticks bite, often include scalp, neck, armpit, groin	No pain, no itching at time of bite. Fever-rash occurs in the week following the bite(s).

' These conditions are contagious

² See pages 50 and 118–20 for more information on chicken pox

SUNBURN

You should never get sunburned. It is not healthy, and leads to premature ageing, wrinkling of the skin and skin cancer.

Sunburn is caused by over-exposure to ultraviolet (UV) light. This can be from the sun, sun-lamps or even from some workplace light sources (e.g., welding arcs). Sunburn results in red, swollen, painful and sometimes blistered skin. Chills, fever, nausea and vomiting can occur if the sunburn is extensive and severe.

The risk for sunburn is increased for:
- Persons with fair skin, blue eyes, and red or blonde hair
- Persons taking some medications including sulpha drugs, tetracyclines and some diuretics (water tablets)
- Persons exposed to industrial UV light sources
- Persons exposed to excessive outdoor sunlight

Sunburn can be prevented by using the following measures:
- Avoid the sun's rays between the hours of 10:00 a.m. and 4:00 p.m.
- Use sunblock with a sun protective factor [SPF] of 15 or more when exposed to the sun. The lighter your skin the higher the SPF number should be. To be effective, sunscreen should be reapplied every hour and after swimming. Make-up is now available with sunscreening protection.
- Wear muted colours such as tan. Brilliant colours and white reflect the sun onto the face.
- Wear a hat when in the sun.

Questions to Ask

Are there any signs, even temporary ones of dehydration, such as:
- Confusion
- Very little or no urine output
- Sunken eyes
- Extreme dryness in the mouth

 YES

NO

Do you have a fever of 39°C (102°F) or higher or have severe pain or blistering with the sunburn?

YES

NO

Self-Care Procedures

- Cool the affected area with clean towels, cloths or gauze dipped in cool water or take a cool bath or shower.
- Take aspirin, paracetamol or ibuprofen to relieve pain and headache and to reduce fever. *Note: Do not give aspirin, or any medication containing salicylates, to children under 12 years of age, unless directed by a doctor, due to its association with Reye's syndrome, a potentially fatal condition.*
- Use an over-the-counter topical steroid cream (1% hydrocortisone if the pain persists. Use it sparingly and not over a large area.

- Rest in a comfortable position, in a cool, quiet room.
- Drink plenty of water to replace fluid loss.
- Avoid using local anaesthetic creams or sprays because they can cause allergic reactions in some people.

VARICOSE VEINS

Varicose veins are swollen and twisted veins that look blue and are close to the surface of the skin. They are unsightly and uncomfortable. Veins bulge, throb and feel heavy. The legs and feet can swell. The skin can itch. Varicose veins may occur in almost any part of your body. They are most often seen in the back of the calf or on the inside of the leg between the groin and the ankle. Haemorrhoids (veins around the anus) are a type of varicose vein. Causes and risk factors for varicose veins include:
- Obesity
- Pregnancy
- Hormonal changes at the menopause
- Activities or hobbies that require standing for a long time
- A family history of varicose veins
- Past vein diseases such as throm-bophlebitis (Inflammation of a vein before a blood clot forms)

Medical treatment is not required for most varicose veins unless problems result, such as severe bleeding caused by injury to the vein.

Surgery can be performed to remove enlarged veins. Sclerotherapy can also be done on smaller veins. This procedure uses a chemical injection into the vein that causes it to close up. Other veins then take over its work. Both of these treatments, however, may bring only temporary success; following either, more varicose veins may develop.

Questions to Ask

Has the varicose vein become swollen, red, very tender or warm to the touch? **YES**

NO

Are varicose veins accompanied by a rash or sores on the leg or near the ankle or have they caused circulation problems in your feet? **YES**

NO

Self-Care Procedures

To relieve and prevent varicose veins:
- Don't cross your legs when sitting.
- Exercise regularly. Walking is a good choice. It improves leg and vein strength.
- Keep your weight down.
- Avoid standing for prolonged periods of time. If your job or hobby requires you to stand, shift your weight from one leg to the other every few minutes.

- Wear elastic support stockings.
- Don't wear clothing or underwear that is tight or constricts your waist, groin or legs.
- Eat high-fibre foods like bran cereals, wholemeal bread, beans, fruit and vegetables to promote regularity. (Constipation contributes to varicose veins.)
- Exercise your legs. (From a sitting position, rotate your feet at the ankles, turning them first clockwise, then anti-clockwise, using a circular motion. Next, extend your legs forward and point your toes to the ceiling, then to the floor. Then, lift your feet off the floor and gently bend your legs backwards and forwards at the knees.)
- Raise your legs when resting.
- Get up and move about every 35 to 45 minutes when travelling by air or even when sitting in an all-day conference. (Opt for an aisle seat in such situations.)

CHAPTER 4
DIGESTIVE PROBLEMS

CONSTIPATION

Constipation is when you have trouble passing stools. Abdominal swelling, straining during bowel movements, hard stools and the feeling of continued fullness even after a bowel movement are also signs of constipation. It can be very uncomfortable, but it usually doesn't signal disease or a serious problem. What factors cause or lead to constipation? A number of things do. These include:
- Not drinking enough fluids
- Not eating enough dietary fibre
- Not being active enough
- Using laxatives over a long period of time
- Taking certain medicines (e.g., painkillers and antidepressant medicines)
- Not going to the toilet when you have the urge to open your bowels
- Medical problems such as haemorrhoids or an under-active thyroid gland

It is important to know that it is not necessary to open your bowels daily. Some people only open their bowels every three or four days and this is normal for them. What is more important is a change in your regular pattern.

The 'cure' for constipation generally consists of correcting the sort of habits that make bowel habits irregular. (See Self-Care Procedures.) You may also need to discuss measures with your doctor about medications and health conditions that could be causing you to be constipated.

Questions to Ask

Do you have any of these problems with the constipation:
- Fever
- Severe abdominal pain (especially located in the lower left section)
- Abdominal bloating
- Weight loss
- Very thin, pencil-like stools or blood seen in the stools

YES

NO

Did you get constipated after taking prescribed or over-the-counter medicines and/or vitamins?

YES

NO

Do you have persistent constipation despite using the Self-Care Procedures listed?

YES

NO

Self-Care Procedures

- Eat foods high in dietary fibre such as bran, wholemeal bread and cereals, fresh fruit and vegetables daily. They serve as natural stool softeners, thanks in part to their fibre content. One type of fibre absorbs water like a sponge, resulting in large, soft masses which are easy to pass.
- Drink plenty of water and other liquids (at least eight glasses a day) to give the fibre plenty of water to absorb.
- Get plenty of exercise, to help your bowels move things along.
- Don't resist the urge to open your bowels or don't put off a trip to the toilet.
- Keep in mind that drugs such as antacids and iron supplements can be constipating, and don't use them if you get constipated easily. (Discuss this with your doctor first.)
- If necessary, for occasional constipation, you may need an over-the-counter stool softener or mild laxative. (Check with your doctor in advance so you'll know what is best for you to take if and when you do get constipated.)

Ask your doctor about the use of 'bulk-forming' laxatives such as Fybogel. You may be able to use these daily, if necessary. Start out slowly and gradually increase how much you take. Also drink plenty of liquids with them. Bloating, cramping or wind may be noticed at first, but these symptoms should go away in a few weeks or less.

Do not use 'stimulant' laxatives such as senna. In the long run, they can make you even more constipated, because your intestines can become lazy and won't work as well on their own. Long-term use of these laxatives can also lead to a mineral imbalance, cause problems with your body's use of other medicines and lower the amount of nutrients you absorb.

DIARRHOEA

Diarrhoea is the frequent passing of watery, loose bowel movements. Almost everyone gets diarrhoea once in a while. Usually, it lasts only a day or two and isn't serious.

Many things can cause diarrhoea:
- Infection by virus, bacteria or parasites
- Food poisoning
- Allergies
- Anxiety
- Too many laxatives
- Certain drugs (For example, many common antibiotics can give you diarrhoea.)
- Diverticulitis (a disease of the bowel)
- Inflammatory bowel disease, usually ulcerative colitis or Crohn's disease

Questions to Ask

If the person with diarrhoea is a baby or child: Does the baby and/or child have any of these problems with the diarrhoea:
- Sunken eyes
- Dry skin and dry mouth
- Dry nappy for more than 3 hours in a baby
- Passing no urine for more than 6 hours in a child
- Feeling weak and tired
- Very fractious
- Weak cry

YES

NO

Does an adult have any of these problems with the diarrhoea:
- Black stools
- Feeling very thirsty and not passing much urine
- Blood in the stool
- Severe pain in the stomach
- Extremely dry mouth

YES

NO

Has the diarrhoea lasted 48 hours or more? And/or does the person have a fever of 38.5°C (101°F) or higher?

YES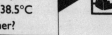

NO

flowchart continued in next column

Are any medicines being taken? (Medicine you take may not be working because of the diarrhoea. Or a medicine may be giving you the diarrhoea.)

YES

NO

If the person is a baby or ill older person, are they getting the diarrhoea more than eight times a day?

YES

NO

Did the person just come back from a trip to another country?

YES

NO

Self-Care Procedures

- Watch out for dehydration.
- Drink plenty of clear liquids. Sucking ice or ice lollies helps, too.
  - Adults or children who are vomiting should take small sips of still drinks regularly, particularly straight after vomiting.
  - Adults who are not vomiting should drink about 3/4 litre (1 pint) an hour unless they are vomiting.
  - Children over two years of age who are not vomiting can drink up to about 2 litres (3 1/2 pints) a day. Ask your doctor for help if the child is thirsty, has cramps, or seems weak or confused.

- Ask your doctor what to give a child under two years of age. At most chemists you can buy powders (e.g., Dioralyte or Rehydrat) to make up into rehydration solutions. These solutions can also be useful for older children or adults.
- Other examples of clear liquids are:
  - Water
  - Clear broth
  - Soft drinks such as colas, 7-Up or Sprite (all of which must be allowed to go flat before being drunk)
  - Weak tea with sugar
  - A mixture of eight level teaspoons of sugar and one level teaspoon of salt with 1 litre ($1^3/_4$ pints) of water
- Don't drink very hot or very cold liquids.
- Don't drink apple juice, as it can worsen diarrhoea, especially in children. Don't drink milk at this time either, as it too can worsen diarrhoea.
- Eat little or no solids the first few days. Jelly is acceptable. It counts as a clear liquid.

When the diarrhoea starts to get better, follow these tips:
- Eat dry biscuits and toast before you try other solid foods.
- Eat small amounts of soft foods like cooked potatoes. Avoid meat, nuts, beans and dairy foods.
- Don't eat high-fibre foods like wholemeal bread or bran cereal.
- Don't eat foods that are hard to digest:
  - Raw fruits and vegetables
  - Fried foods
  - Sweets

- Don't drink coffee (it's hard on your stomach).
- Don't exercise too hard until the diarrhoea is gone.
- For adults and children over 12, you can try an over-the-counter drug containing loperamide (e.g., Imodium).

Follow these tips to avoid spreading infection:
- Wash your hands with soap after you use the toilet.
- Wash your hands before you cook.
- Don't share towels with others.
- Dry your hands with paper towels and throw the towels away.

FLATULENCE

Flatulence may be perfectly natural and something that everyone has at one time or another, but if you have more than your share, it's a major annoyance.

Where does all that wind come from? Often, it comes from swallowing air. It's also generated by intestinal bacteria that produce carbon dioxide and hydrogen (both odourless, by the way) in the course of breaking down carbohydrates and proteins in the food you eat. The minute quantities of other, more pungent gases gives flatus its characteristic odour. Eating certain foods, like peas, beans and certain grains produces noticeably more wind than eating other foods. All roughage in the diet will produce flatulence. A high-roughage diet, especially, will do this. When increasing dietary fibre in your diet, do so gradually.

This will lessen the increase of flatus. Wind may signal a variety of other problems worth looking into:
- Lactose intolerance (inability properly to digest milk, cheese and other dairy products)
- Bacterial overgrowth in the intestines (often caused by certain antibiotics)
- Abnormal muscle contraction in the colon.

Questions to Ask

Is the flatulence accompanied by severe steady pain in the upper abdomen, nausea and vomiting, or yellowing of the skin or eyes? **YES**

NO

Has the flatulence occurred only after taking a prescribed antibiotic? **YES**

NO

Self-Care Procedures

Common sense says eliminating food items that often cause wind (or eating them in small quantities) can go a long way towards reducing excess flatulence. Well-known offenders include:
- Apples
- Apricots

- Aubergines
- Beans (dried, cooked)
- Bran
- Broccoli
- Brussels sprouts
- Cabbage
- Carrots
- Cauliflower
- Dairy products (for people allergic to lactose)
- Nuts
- Onions
- Peaches
- Pears
- Popcorn
- Prunes
- Raisins
- Soya beans

(Eliminate or go easy on only the foods that affect you personally. All the foods listed are good sources of nutrients, so they should not be cut out altogether.)
- Keep a list of all the foods you eat for a few days and note when and the number of times you have wind. If you notice that you have excess wind after drinking milk, for example, try cutting down on it or eliminate it from your diet. See if the flatulence persists. Do the same for other suspect foods.
- If you are lactose-intolerant use lactose-reduced dairy foods.
- Avoid swallowing air at mealtimes by eating more slowly.

HEARTBURN

Heartburn has nothing to do with your heart. The pain comes from stomach acid that travels up into your oesophagus (the tube that connects your throat to your stomach). The oesophagus passes behind the breastbone alongside the heart, so the irritation that takes place there feels like a burning feeling in the heart. All these things can cause heartburn:

- Taking aspirin, ibuprofen, arthritis medicine or steroids
- Eating heavy meals
- Eating too fast
- Eating foods like chocolate, garlic, onions, peppermint, tomatoes or citrus fruits
- Lying down after a meal
- Smoking after eating
- Drinking coffee, even decaffeinated coffee
- Drinking alcohol
- Pregnancy
- Wearing tight clothing
- Being extremely overweight
- Swallowing too much air
- Stress
- Hiatus hernia (a bulging of the upper part of the stomach through the diaphragm)

Questions to Ask

Does your chest feel tight? Does the tightness go to your neck, jaw or arm? Are you sweating or short of breath? Does your pain get worse with exertion? Are you suffering from nausea? **YES**

NO

Are you vomiting anything black or red in colour? **YES**

NO

Are your stools tar-like and black in colour? **YES**

NO

Do you also have pain that goes through your back or a gripping pain in the upper abdomen? **YES**

NO

Is it hard for you to swallow? **YES**

NO

Have you had the heartburn many times over the last three days? **YES**

NO

Self-Care Procedures

Stay away from foods you know give you heartburn. Try these tips, too:

- Don't smoke. It encourages heartburn.
- Sit straight. Stand up or walk around often. Don't bend over or lie down after you eat.
- Raise the head of your bed by about 15 cm (6 in) if you get heartburn at night. You can do this by putting blocks between the mattress and the base of the bed.
- Keep your weight down. The top of your stomach can push up through your diaphragm if you're overweight. This can happen to pregnant women, too.
- Don't wear clothes that are tight around your stomach, like girdles.
- Eat small meals.
- Don't eat anything for at least three hours before going to bed.
- Try an over-the-counter preparation to counter indigestion. There are two main types:
  - Antacids (e.g., Rennies, Gaviscon) as either tablets or liquid. These neutralize stomach acid. Talk to your doctor before taking them if you have kidney disease, heart disease or high blood pressure.
  - Acid suppressors (e.g., Tagamet, Zantac). These stop the stomach making acid in the first place. They are very effective but if symptoms return when you have finished the course you must consult your doctor before taking any more.
  - Don't take baking soda. (Another name for baking soda is bicarbonate of soda or 'bicarb' for short.) It seems to help at first, but the acid comes back worse later.
- Don't smoke. It encourages heartburn.
- Don't drink through straws or bottles with narrow mouths.
- If you need to take aspirin, ibuprofen, arthritis medicines or cortisone, take them with food or milk.

Call your doctor if you have no relief after using Self-Care Procedures.

HAEMORRHOIDS

Haemorrhoids are veins in the wall of the rectum or around the anus that are dilated or swollen. They are caused by repeated pressure in the rectal or anal veins. This pressure usually results from repeated straining to pass bowel movements. Rarely they result from benign or malignant tumours of the abdomen or rectum. The risk of getting haemorrhoids increases with:

- Constipation
- Low dietary fibre intake
- Pregnancy and delivery
- Obesity

Symptoms of haemorrhoids include:

- Rectal bleeding
- Rectal tenderness and/or itching
- Uncomfortable, painful bowel movements, especially with straining
- A lump that can be felt in the anus
- A mucus discharge after a bowel movement

Haemorrhoids are common and most people have some bleeding from them once in a while. Though annoying and uncomfortable, haemorrhoids are seldom a serious health problem. However, they can occur with other anal and rectal conditions which can be serious. Anyone who experiences new rectal bleeding should see their doctor to confirm the diagnosis of haemorrhoids.

If you already know you have haemorrhoids you should seek medical advice if you have:
- Excessive bleeding
- Severe pain lasting more than 48 hours
- Any change in the symptoms usually associated with your haemorrhoids

If symptoms of haemorrhoids are not relieved with Self-Care Procedures listed or with time, medical treatment may be necessary. This includes:
- Cryosurgery which freezes the affected tissue
- Injecting a chemical into an internal haemorrhoid to shrink it
- Electrical or laser heat or infrared light to destroy the haemorrhoids
- Surgery called haemorrhoidectomy. One type, which requires general anaesthesia, cuts out the haemorrhoids. Another, called ligation, uses rubber bands that are placed tightly over the base of each haemorrhoid causing them to wither away.

Questions to Ask

Do you have severe rectal bleeding that is continuous or associated with weakness or dizziness? **YES**

NO

Do you have rectal bleeding:
- Without bowel movements
- That is heavy, dark red or turns brown
- That lasts longer than two weeks despite using self-care procedures

YES

NO

Do you have a hard lump where a haemorrhoid used to be? **YES**

NO

Do you have severe pain lasting longer than 48 hours? Or do you have moderate pain lasting longer than a week? **YES**

NO

63

Self-Care Procedures

To produce easily passed bowel movements:
- Drink plenty of water and other fluids: at least 1½ to 2 litres (2 to 3 pints) a day.
- Eat foods with good sources of dietary fibre such as whole grain or bran cereals and breads, fresh vegetables and fruit.
- Eat prunes and/or drink prune juice.
- Add bran to your foods, if necessary (about three to four tablespoons per day).
- Exercise regularly.
- Pass a bowel movement as soon as you feel the urge. If you wait and the urge goes away, your stool could become dry and be harder to pass.
- Lose weight if you are overweight.
- Don't strain to pass a stool.
- Keep the anal area clean.
- Take warm baths.
- Check with your doctor about using over-the-counter products such as:
  - Stool softeners
  - Zinc oxide preparations such as Anusol. But avoid preparations containing local anaesthetics which can cause skin sensitivity.
  - Medicated suppositories
- Don't sit too much because it can restrict blood flow around the anal area.
- Don't sit too long on the toilet.
- For itching or pain, put cold compresses on the anus for 10 minutes up to four times a day.

VOMITING AND NAUSEA

Vomiting is when you actually expel your stomach contents via your mouth.

Nausea is when you feel like you're going to vomit. Here are some common causes of nausea and vomiting:
- Viral infections such as gastroenteritis (You can get diarrhoea, too.)
- Morning sickness in pregnant women
- Some medications
- Food poisoning
- Eating or drinking too much

Some serious problems also cause vomiting, but there are almost always other symptoms as well. Examples of such problems are:
- Appendicitis
- Acute glaucoma
- Stomach ulcers
- Hepatitis (inflammation of the liver)
- Meningitis (inflammation of membranes that cover the brain and spinal cord)
- Brain tumours

Questions to Ask

Do you have any of these problems along with the vomiting:
- Stiff neck, fever and headache
- Black or bloody vomit
- Severe pain in and around one eye
- Blurred eyesight
- A head injury that happened in the last 48 hours

YES

NO

flowchart continued on next page

64

Dehydration is when your body loses too much water. Do you have any of these signs of dehydration:
• Feeling confused
• Very little or no urine
• Sunken eyes
• Wrinkled or saggy skin

YES

NO

Do you have very bad stomach pain? Does it last for more than two hours? Does it keep hurting even after you vomit?

YES

NO

Do the whites of your eyes or your skin look yellow?

YES

NO

Do you have any of these problems:
• Burning or stinging feeling when you pass urine
• Passing urine a lot more often than usual
• Bloody or cloudy urine
• Pain in your abdomen or over your bladder

YES

NO

flowchart continued in next column

Have you been vomiting up for more than 12 hours without getting better?

YES

NO

In a small child, has the vomiting lasted more than four hours?

YES

NO

Are you vomiting medicine that is necessary for you to take? (Birth control pills and high blood pressure pills are examples.)

YES

NO

Self-Care Procedures

• Don't eat solid food until you stop vomiting.
• Drink clear liquids at room temperature (not too cold or too hot). Take small sips. Drink only one to two ounces at a time. Water, colas and ginger ale are good. Stir any carbonated drinks to get all the bubbles out before sipping them. Don't drink alcohol. Suck on ice cubes if you can't take anything else.
• After you stop vomiting, try eating dry biscuits or toast.
• Don't smoke.
• Don't take aspirin.
• Call your doctor if you don't get better or if the vomiting returns.

CHAPTER 5
MUSCLE AND BONE PROBLEMS

BACKACHES

Most backaches come from strained muscles in the lower back. Other causes include back injuries such as a slipped or herniated disc, arthritis or osteoporosis. The goals of treatment are to treat the cause of the backache, relieve the pain, promote healing and avoid re-injury.

How to Avoid Back Pain

Lifting causes a lot of backaches. Here are some lifting Do's and Don'ts to help you avoid straining your back.

Do's:
• Wear good shoes with low heels, not sandals or high heels.
• Stand close to the thing you want to lift.
• Plant your feet squarely, shoulder width apart.
• Bend at the knees, not at the waist. Keep your knees bent as you lift.
• Pull in your stomach and buttocks.
• Keep your back as straight as you can.
• Hold the object close to your body.
• Lift slowly.
• Let your legs carry the weight.
• Get help or use a trolley to move something very heavy.

Don'ts:
• Don't lift if your back hurts.
• Don't lift if you have a history of back trouble.
• Don't lift something that's too heavy.
• Don't lift heavy things over your head.
• Don't lift anything heavy if you're not steady on your feet.
• Don't bend at the waist to pick something up.
• Don't arch your back when you lift or carry.
• Don't lift too fast or with a jerk.
• Don't twist your back when you are holding something. Turn your whole body, from head to toe.
• Don't lift something heavy with one hand and something light with the other. Balance the load.
• Don't try to lift one thing while you hold something else. For example, don't try to pick up a child while you are holding a grocery bag. Put the bag down, or lift the bag and the child at the same time.

Questions to Ask

Is the back pain extreme and felt across the upper back (not just on one side) and did it come on suddenly (within about 15 minutes) with no apparent reason such as an injury or back strain? **YES**

NO

Did the pain start inside your chest and move to the upper back? **YES**

NO

Was the back pain sudden with a cracking sound? **YES**

NO

Did the pain come after a recent fall, injury or violent movement to the back, and are you having difficulty moving your arm or leg? Do you also have numbness or tingling in your legs, feet, toes, arms or hands and/or loss of bladder or bowel control? **YES**

NO

Did the pain come on all of a sudden after being unable to get about for a long time, or are you over 60 years old? **YES**

NO

flowchart continued in next column

Is the pain severe (but not a result of a fall or injury to the back), and has it lasted for more than five to seven days, or is there also a sense of weakness, numbness or tingling in the feet or toes? **YES**

NO

Does the pain travel down the legs below the knee? **YES**

NO

Does it hurt more when you move, cough, sneeze, lift or strain? **YES**

NO

Does it hurt, burn or itch when you pass urine? Do you have fever or vomiting with the pain? Do you have to go to the toilet more often? Does your urine smell or have blood in it? **YES**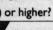

NO

Is the pain felt on one side of the small of your back, just above the waist, and do you feel sick and have a fever of 38.5°C (101°F) or higher? **YES**

NO

flowchart continued on next page

Do you also have any of
the following:
* Joint stiffness and pain
* Redness, heat or
  swelling in affected joints
* Cracking or grating
  sounds with joint
  movement

YES

NO

Self-Care Procedures

Bed rest – Resting the back can help
treat the pain and avoid re-injury. Resting
doesn't have to be in bed, but lying down
takes pressure off your back so it can heal
faster. Up to three days of bed rest is
usually recommended. Your back muscles
can get weak if you stay in bed longer
than that. To make the most of rest:
* When you need to get up from bed,
  move slowly, roll on your side and swing
  your legs to the floor. Push off the bed
  with your arms.
* Get comfortable when you are lying,
  standing and sitting. For example, when
  you lie on your back, keep your upper
  back flat but your hips and knees bent.
  Keep your feet flat on the bed. Tip your
  hips down and up until you find the best
  spot.
* Take pressure off your lower back. Put a
  pillow under your knees or lie on your
  side with your knees bent.

Cold treatment – Cold helps treat
bruises and swelling. You can make a cold
pack by wrapping ice in a towel. Use the
cold pack for 20 minutes, then take it off
for 20 minutes. Do this repeatedly for
two to three hours a day. Lie on your
back with your knees bent and put the
ice pack under your lower back. Start as
soon as you hurt your back. Keep doing it
for three to four days.

Heat treatment – Heat makes blood
flow, which helps healing. But don't use
heat on a back strain until three to four
days after the injury occurred. If you use
heat sooner, it can make the pain and
swelling worse. Use a heating pad, a
wrapped hot-water bottle, hot
compresses, a heat lamp, hot baths or
hot showers. Use heat for 20 minutes,
then take the heat off for 20 minutes.
Do this up to three hours a day. Be
careful not to burn yourself.

Massage – Massage won't cure a
backache, but it can loosen tight muscles.

Braces or corsets – Braces and corsets
support your back and keep you from
moving it too much. They do what strong
back muscles do, but they won't make
your back stronger and may make the
muscles weaker.

Pain relief – Take aspirin or ibuprofen
for pain. *Note: Do not give aspirin, or any
medication containing salicylates, to children
under 12 years of age, unless directed by a
doctor, due to its association with Reye's
syndrome, a potentially fatal condition.*

Paracetamol will help the pain but not the swelling.

Don't overdo it after taking a painkiller. You can hurt your back more and then it will take longer to heal.

More Tips

• After two to three days of resting your back, try some mild stretching exercises to make stomach and back muscles stronger. Exercise in the morning and afternoon. (Always ask your doctor before starting an exercise programme.)

• Don't sit in one place longer than you need to. It strains your lower back.

• Sleep on a firm but not hard mattress.

• Never sleep on your stomach. Sleep on your back or side, with your knees bent.

• If your back pain is chronic or doesn't get better on its own, see your doctor. He or she can evaluate your needs. A referral may be given to a physiotherapist.

BROKEN BONES

Bones break when subjected to excessive force. An arm, leg or finger that is twisted in the wrong direction, hit too hard or crushed by accident can splinter and snap.

You may think that the body's 206 bones are as dry and lifeless as dead tree branches. Not so. Bones are made up of living tissue. New bone is added and old bone is broken down daily. This non-stop process continues from before we are born until we are about 35 years old, after which our bones gradually start to thin as the building process slows down.

There are different kinds of broken bones. Some are called 'greenstick' fractures because on the X-ray, the barely visible fracture resembles the pattern of a very young splintered twig. They occur particularly in children.

Other breaks are more complicated. Sometimes the bone protrudes through the skin and is called a compound fracture. In other cases, the bone may separate partially or completely from the other half. Bones can also break in more than one place.

Bones in children are more pliable and resilient than those in adults. In most cases, children's bones are still growing, especially the long bones of their arms and legs. Damage to the ends of these bones should be monitored carefully because of the risk of stunting the bone's growth.

Bones in some elderly people become dangerously thin with age. Many post-menopausal women and some elderly men suffer from osteoporosis, a condition in which the bones gradually become thinner. The bones in people with osteoporosis become brittle and break easily. The female hormone oestrogen protects women from osteoporosis until they reach the menopause. Hormone replacement therapy (HRT) can help after the menopause.

Broken bones need immediate treatment. Not only are they intensely painful, but unless properly cared for, broken bones may cause future deformities and limited movement.

Prevention

Make sure you and your child wear appropriate protective equipment such as elbow pads, knee pads and a helmet during sporting and recreational events.

Check that everyone in the car is wearing a seat belt. Don't start the engine until everyone's seat belt is fastened.

If you or your child likes to use roller-blades, these tips may prevent injury:

- Always wear a helmet, elbow and knee pads and wrist guards.
- Skate on smooth, paved surfaces.
- Avoid skating at night.
- Learn how to stop.

If you are a post-menopausal woman, talk to your doctor about hormone replacement therapy and:

- Exercise. Moderate weight-bearing exercise such as walking, aerobics and dancing increases bone mass.
- Eat calcium-rich foods such as low-fat milk products, sardines, broccoli and calcium-fortified foods such as juices, cereals and bread.
- Take calcium supplements if advised by your doctor.
- If you smoke, stop. If you drink alcohol, limit the amount.

Questions to Ask

Is the person showing these signs of shock:
- Fainting
- Sweating, dizziness, increased thirst, rapid, weak pulse rate
- Cold, pale and clammy skin

YES

NO

Does the person have:
- A broken bone in the pelvis or thigh
- Cold, blue skin under the fracture
- Numbness below the fracture

YES

NO

If a rib is cracked, is the person also suffering shortness of breath? Is there any deformity at the fracture site? Is the pain so severe the person is unable to use the injured limb normally?

YES

NO

Is there a lot of bleeding and bruising around the injury?

YES

NO

Is the injury still painful after 48 hours?

YES

NO

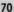

Self-Care Procedures

All broken bones require a doctor's attention. Do not try to set a broken bone yourself or try to push a protruding bone back under the skin. However, you may need to immobilize the injured limb until you get medical attention.

- A splint is a good way to immobilize the affected area, reduce pain and prevent shock.
  - Effective splints can be made from rolled-up newspapers and magazines, an umbrella, a stick, a cane and rolled-up blankets. Place this type of item around the injury and gently hold it in place with a belt, tie or strip of cloth. The general rule is to splint the joints above and below the fracture.
  - Lightly tape or tie an injured leg to the uninjured one, putting padding between the legs, if possible. Tape an injured arm to the chest, if the elbow is bent, or to the side if the elbow is straight, placing padding between the body and the arm.
  - For a broken arm, make a sling out of a triangular piece of cloth. Place the forearm in it and tie the ends around the neck so the arm is resting at a 90° angle.
  - Check the pulse in the splinted limb. If you cannot find it, the splint is too tight and must be loosened at once.
  - Check for swelling, numbness, tingling or a blue tinge to the skin. Any of these signs indicate the splint is too tight and must be immediately loosened to prevent permanent injury.
  - Keep the person quiet to avoid moving the injured area.

- Apply ice to the injured area to help reduce swelling and inflammation.
- Take ibuprofen to reduce pain and swelling. Paracetamol will help the pain but not the swelling.

SHOULDER AND NECK PAIN

Shoulder and neck pain is a common condition. Driving a golf ball, cleaning windows or reaching for a jar can strain and injure shoulder muscles and tendons, especially in people who are out of condition. Fortunately, this discomfort rarely suggests a serious condition. Causes of shoulder and neck pain include:

- Poor posture and/or unnatural sleeping positions. Sleeping on a soft mattress can give you a stiff neck the next morning.
- Tension and stress. When you feel tense, the muscles around your neck can go into spasm.
- Tendinitis, inflammation of a tendon, the tissue that connects muscles to bone. Left untreated, tendinitis can turn into 'frozen shoulder', a stiff, painful condition that may limit your ability to use your shoulder.
- Bursitis, an inflammation of the sac (bursa) that encases the shoulder joint. Bursitis can be caused by injury, infection, overuse, arthritis or gout.
- Osteoarthritis in the neck. Unlike rheumatoid arthritis, osteoarthritis can develop in joints subjected to normal wear-and-tear as we age or from repeated injuries. Ageing can cause the

joints to wear out, producing bony spurs that can press on nerves and cause pain.

- Accidents and falls. Collarbones can break after falls or road traffic accidents.
- Road traffic accidents. You can sustain a whiplash injury when your vehicle is hit from behind.
- Pinched nerve. Arthritis or an injury to your neck can pinch a nerve in your neck. Pain from a pinched nerve usually runs down the arm and one side only.

Sometimes shoulder and neck pain signals serious medical problems, especially with other symptoms such as stiff neck, sudden and severe headache, dizziness, chest pain or pressure and/or loss of consciousness.

Prevention

- Stretching and strengthening routines, especially before exercising, helps prevent tendinitis. So can using the correct equipment and following the proper technique.
- Avoid injuries to the shoulder by wearing seat belts and having head restraints in vehicles and using protective clothing and equipment during sporting events.
- Avoid vigorous exercise unless you are fit. If you are out of condition, start to strengthen your muscles gradually and slowly increase exercise intensity.
- Don't sleep on your stomach. You are likely to twist your neck in this position.
- Sleep on a firm mattress. Use a thinner pillow or none at all if you have pain when you wake up.

Keep the muscles in your shoulders strong and flexible to prevent injury. These exercises can help:

- Stretch the back of your shoulder by reaching with one arm under your chin and across the opposite shoulder, gently push the arm towards your collarbone with the other hand. Hold for 15 seconds. Repeat five times, then switch sides.
- Raise one arm and bend it behind your head to touch the opposite shoulder. Use the other hand to pull the elbow gently towards the opposite shoulder. Hold for 15 seconds. Repeat five times, then switch sides.
- Holding light weights, lift your arms out horizontally and slightly forward. Keeping your thumbs towards the floor, slowly lower your arms halfway, then return to shoulder level. Repeat 10 times.
- Sit straight in a chair. Flex your neck slowly forwards and try to touch your chin to your chest. Hold for 10 seconds and go back to the starting position. Repeat five times.
- Sit straight in a chair. Look straight ahead. Slowly tilt your head to the right, trying to touch your right ear to your right shoulder. Do not raise your shoulder to meet your ear. Hold for 10 seconds and straighten your head. Repeat five times on this side and then on your left side.

Questions to Ask

Along with the shoulder and neck pain are you:
- Feeling pressure in your chest, especially on the left side
- Short of breath or having trouble breathing
- Nauseated and/or vomiting
- Sweating
- Anxious
- Having irregular heartbeats

YES

NO

Did you experience a serious injury that caused shoulder and/or neck pain that is not going away and/or is getting worse?

YES

NO

Do you have a stiff neck along with a severe headache from nausea or vomiting?

YES

NO

flowchart continued in next column

Do you have any of the following:
- Severe or persistent pain, swelling, spasms or a deformity in your shoulder
- A shoulder that is painful and stiff with reduced ability to move it
- Stabbing pain, numbness or tingling
- Pain, tenderness and limited motion in the shoulder

YES

NO

Is the shoulder pain severe, interfering with your sleep? Is the shoulder stiff in the morning, swollen, tender or hard to move?

YES

NO

Self-Care Procedures

Unfortunately, no matter how careful people are, injuries do occur. Injured tendons, muscles and ligaments in any part of the body can take a long time to heal. Longer, in fact, than a broken bone. Don't ignore the aches and pains. Studies show that exercising before an injury has healed may not only worsen it, but may greatly increase the chance for re-injury.

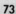

Put the arm with the injured shoulder in a sling when you take the person to the doctor.

Treating tendinitis – Taking over-the-counter pain relievers such as aspirin or ibuprofen eases the pain and reduces inflammation. Paracetamol eases muscle soreness but does not help with inflammation. *Note: Do not give aspirin, or any medication containing salicylates, to children under 12 years of age, unless directed by a doctor, due to its association with Reye's syndrome, a potentially fatal condition.*

Although the pain of tendinitis can linger for weeks, it usually disappears in a few days if given proper treatment:

• Rest the injured shoulder. Rest prevents further inflammation, giving the tendon a chance to heal. Resume your activities only after the pain is completely gone.

• Apply ice to the injured area as soon as possible. Immediately putting ice on the injury helps to speed recovery because it not only relieves pain, but also slows blood flow, reducing internal bleeding and swelling.

• Put ice cubes or crushed ice in a heavy plastic bag with a little water. You can also use a bag of frozen vegetables. Wrap the ice pack in a towel before placing it on the injured areas.

• Apply the ice pack to the injured shoulder for 10 to 20 minutes. Reapply it every two hours and for the next 48 hours during the times you are not sleeping.

The swelling is usually eased within 48 hours. Once the swelling is gone, apply heat to speed up healing, help relieve pain, relax muscles and reduce joint stiffness.

• Use a heated pad set on low or medium or a heat lamp for dry heat. Or use a wrapped hot-water bottle, heat pack or hot, damp towel wrapped around the injured area for moist heat. (Damp heat should be no warmer than 40.5°C/105°F.)

• Apply heat to the injured area for 20 to 30 minutes, two to three times a day.

Topical preparations of drugs like ibuprofen can relieve pain and speed up healing in some cases. (Ask your pharmacist for advice.)

Liniments and balms also relieve the discomfort of sore muscles. They provide a cooling or warming sensation. Although these ointments only mask the pain of sore muscles and do nothing to promote healing, massaging them into the shoulder increases blood flow to help relax the muscles.

Treating bursitis – Arthritis or any prolonged use of a joint can cause the pain and discomfort of bursitis. Fortunately, these flare-ups can be controlled by:

• Applying ice packs to the sore shoulders

• Taking a hot shower, using a heat lamp, applying a hot compress or heated pad to the affected shoulder or rubbing the area with a deep-heating liniment.

Treating neck pain from whiplash injuries or pinched nerves – Always see a doctor if your motor vehicle is ever hit from the rear because the accident can cause a whiplash injury. The recommended treatment for whiplash injuries usually consists of using hot and cold packs, massage, exercises, sometimes a soft collar and pain-relieving medications such as aspirin, paracetamol or ibuprofen. Once your symptoms subside, you can resume normal activity. *Note: Do not give aspirin, or any medication containing salicylates, to children under 12 years of age, unless directed by a doctor, due to its association with Reye's syndrome, a potentially fatal condition.*

After first checking with your doctor, you can ease neck discomfort by:

- Resting as much as possible by lying on your back – not sitting up
- Using cold and hot packs. See how to use them in the section on treating tendinitis.
- Improving your posture. When sitting, select a chair with a straight back and push your buttocks into the chair's back. When standing, pull in your chin and stomach.
- Using a cervical (neck) pillow or roll a hand towel and place it under your neck
- Avoiding activities that may aggravate your injuries
- Covering your neck with a scarf in cold weather.
- Practising some of the stretching and strengthening exercises listed under Prevention.

Dealing with arthritis and osteoporosis – See the section on arthritis on page 185 and the section on osteoporosis on page 206 for information on these conditions.

SPORTS INJURIES

Common sports injuries include twisted ankles, painful joints, and stiff, sore muscles. If you continue to exercise when injured, further damage can leave you laid up for weeks or months. 'Break a leg' means good luck only in the theatre world. Take care to avoid injury when exercising.

Prevention

Common sense can prevent many sports injuries. The top six injuries and ways to prevent them are:

Knee injury
- Avoid looking at your knees when standing or moving.
- Do not bend your knees past 90° when doing half knee bends.
- Avoid twisting your knees by keeping your feet flat as much as possible (during stretches).
- Use softest surface available.
- Wear proper shoes with soft, flexible soles.
- When jumping, land with your knees bent.

Muscle soreness (a symptom of having worked out too hard or too long)
- Do warm-up exercises (e.g., those that stretch the muscles before your activity), not only for vigorous activities like running, but also even for less vigorous ones such as golf.
- Don't overdo it.

In vigorous activities, go through a cooling-down period. Spend five minutes doing the activity at a slower pace. For example, after a run, you should walk or walk/jog for five minutes so your pulse drops gradually.

Blisters (due to poor fitting shoes or socks)
- Wear shoes and socks that fit well (the widest area of your foot should match the widest area of the shoe. You should also be able to wiggle your toes with the shoe on in both a sitting and standing position). The inner seams of the shoe should not rub against areas of your feet.
- Apply protective taping, if necessary.

Stitch (sharp pain felt underneath the rib cage)
- Don't eat or drink two hours prior to exercise.
- Do proper breathing by raising abdominal muscles as you breathe in.
- Don't 'work through pain'. Stop activity, then walk slowly.

Shin splints (mild to severe ache in the front of the lower leg)
- Strengthen muscles in this region.
- Keep calves well-stretched.
- When using an indoor track, don't always run in the same direction.

Achilles tendon pain (caused by a stretch, tear or irritation to the tendon that connects the calf muscles to the back of the heel)
- Do warm-up stretching exercises before the activity. Stretch the Achilles tendon area and hold that position. Don't bounce.
- Wear proper-fitting shoes that provide shock absorption and stability. Avoid running shoes that are too high at the back.
- Avoid running on hard surfaces like asphalt and concrete.
- Run on flat surfaces instead of uphill. Running uphill aggravates the stress put on the Achilles tendon.

Questions to Ask

Do you have numbness and inability to move the injured body part or a noticeable deformity of the extremity? **YES**

 NO

Are any of these problems present:
- More than mild pain and swelling
- Blue discoloration of the skin **YES**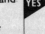

 NO

76

Self-Care Procedures

At the first sign of serious discomfort or pain, stop what you're doing and apply R.I.C.E.: rest, ice, compression, and elevation. By following this easy-to-remember formula, you can avoid further injury and speed recovery.

R Rest the injured area for 24 to 48 hours.

I Ice the area for five to 20 minutes every hour for the first 48 to 72 hours, or until the area no longer looks or feels hot.

C Compress the area by wrapping it tightly with an elastic bandage for 30 minutes, then unwrap it for 15 minutes. Begin wrapping from the point farthest from the heart (distally) and wrap towards the centre of the body (proximally). Repeat several times.

E Elevate the area to reduce swelling. Prop it up to keep it elevated while you sleep.

Also, doctors recommend taking aspirin or ibuprofen to reduce inflammation and pain. *Note: Do not give aspirin, or any medication containing salicylates, to children under 12 years of age, unless directed by a doctor, due to its association with Reye's syndrome, a potentially fatal condition.*

Once the injured area begins to heal, do M.S.A. techniques. M.S.A. stands for movement, strength and alternate activities.

M Movement – Work at establishing a full range of movement as soon as possible after an injury. This will help maintain flexibility during healing and prevent the scar tissue formed by the injury from limiting future performance.

S Strength – Gradually strengthen the injured area once the inflammation is controlled and a range of movement is re-established.

A Alternative Activities – Do regular exercise using activities that do not strain the injured part. This should be started a few days after the injury, even though the injured part is still healing.

SPRAINS AND STRAINS

Sprains and strains happen when you overstretch or tear a tissue between muscles and bones. Sprains and strains hurt and swell up. People often get sprains and strains when they fall, twist an arm or leg, play sports or push their bodies too hard.

How to Avoid Sprains and Strains

Here are some everyday tips:
• Clear ice from paths and pavements in winter.
• Wear shoes and boots with non-slip soles.
• Put handrails on stairs at home.
• Use rubber mats or strips in baths and shower cubicles. A support bar is a good idea, too.

- Make sure there are light switches near the doors in your house. Make sure outside doors and steps are lit at night.
- Put a night-light in the hallway between the bedroom and bathroom.
- Don't leave shoes, toys, tools or other things where people can trip over them.
- Clean floors with non-slip wax. Secure carpet to the floor.
- Make sure rugs have non-slip backing.
- Be careful when you use a ladder. Make sure it's steady. The ladder should be tall enough that you don't have to stand on the top three steps.

Here are some tips for preventing sports injuries:
- Start slowly. Begin an exercise programme doing things that are easy for you. Build up gradually.
- Warm up your muscles with slow, easy stretches before you exercise. You should do this for all kinds of sports. Don't overdo it. If muscles or joints start to hurt, ease up.
- Cool down after hard exercise. Slow down for about five minutes (e.g., five minutes of walking after running).
- Wear shoes that fit you and the exercise you do.

For more tips to avoid strains and sprains, see 'The Do's and Don'ts of Lifting' on page 66.

What to Do for a Sprain or Strain

What should you do for a sprain or strain? That depends on how bad it is. Self-care may work. But you may need a doctor's help for a very bad sprain. He or she may put a cast on the sprain.

Questions to Ask

Did you hurt yourself in a road accident or fall from a high place? YES

NO

Do you note any of these signs:
- A bone sticking out
- A crookedness or wrong shape to the injured body part
- A grating sound from the bones in that part
- A loss of feeling in the injured body part
- An inability to move the injured body part or put weight on it

YES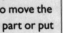

NO

Is the skin blue around the injury? Does the skin feel cold and numb? YES

NO

flowchart continued on next page

Do you note any of these signs:

- The skin around the injury turns blue and/or feels cold and numb
- There is bad pain and swelling
- It hurts to press along the bone
- The pain is getting worse

YES

NO

Call your doctor if the sprain or strain doesn't start to get better after four days.

Self-Care Procedures

Stop what you're doing as soon as you feel the sprain or strain. Then use R.I.C.E. to get better. (See R.I.C.E. in the section 'Sports Injuries' on page 77.)
More tips:

- Take aspirin, ibuprofen or naproxen sodium every four hours for pain and swelling. *Note: Do not give aspirin, or any medication containing salicylates, to children under 12 years of age, unless directed by a doctor, due to its association with Reye's syndrome, a potentially fatal condition.*
- Remove your rings right away if you sprain your finger, hand or wrist. (If you don't and your fingers swell up, someone may have to cut the rings off.)
- Use a walking stick in the opposite hand if you have a badly sprained ankle. It will help keep the weight off the injured ankle so it can heal.

CHAPTER 6
OTHER HEALTH PROBLEMS

ANAEMIA

Are you tired and weak? Does the inside of your lower eyelid look pale? You may be anaemic. But what does that mean?

It means that either your red blood cells or the amount of haemoglobin (oxygen-carrying protein) in your red blood cells is low.

Iron-deficiency anaemia is the most common form of anaemia, affecting perhaps as many as 20 per cent of women of child-bearing age (compared to only 2 per cent of men). The main cause is blood lost during menstruation. But eating too few iron-rich foods or not absorbing enough iron can make the problem worse.

The recommended daily allowance for iron ranges from 10 milligrams for infants to between 30 and 60 milligrams for pregnant women. Yet many females between the ages of 12 and 50 (those at highest risk for iron-deficiency anaemia) have been found to obtain only about half of what they need. Pregnancy, breast-feeding a baby, and blood loss from the gastrointestinal tract (either due to ulcers or cancer) can all deplete the body's iron stores. Anyone, young or old, who has a poor diet is at risk from iron-deficiency anaemia.

Another type of anaemia, sometimes called folic acid deficiency anaemia, occurs when folic acid levels are low, usually due to inadequate dietary intake (common in pregnancy) or to faulty absorption.

Other less-common forms of anaemia include pernicious anaemia (inability of the body to absorb vitamin B_{12} properly), sickle-cell disease (an inherited disorder) and thalassaemia (also inherited).

Alcohol, certain drugs and some chronic diseases can also cause anaemia.

Questions to Ask

Do you have blood in your stools or urine or have black, tar-like stools with these problems:
- Light-headedness
- Weakness
- Shortness of breath
- Severe abdominal pain

 YES

NO

Are you dizzy when you stand up or when you exert yourself?

 YES

NO

Do you have ringing in your ears?

 YES

NO

flowchart continued on next page

For women:
- Do you have menstrual bleeding between periods?
- Has menstrual bleeding been heavy for several months?
- Do you normally bleed seven days or more every month?
- Do you suspect that you are pregnant?

YES

NO

Have symptoms of anaemia (paleness, tiredness, listlessness and weakness) persisted for at least two weeks?

YES

NO

Self-Care Procedures

If you have been diagnosed as suffering from anaemia, the first step is for your doctor to pinpoint the cause. If it's due to a poor diet, you're in luck: Iron-deficiency anaemia is not only the most common form of anaemia, it's the easiest to correct if it's related to menstruation or deficiencies in diet. Folic acid vitamin supplements may also be necessary.

You may need to:
- Eat more foods that are good sources of iron. Concentrate on green, leafy vegetables; lean, red meat; poultry; fish; wheatgerm; dried fruit and iron-fortified cereals.
- Boost your iron absorption. Foods high in vitamin C (e.g., citrus fruits, tomatoes and strawberries help your body absorb iron from food). And red meat not only supplies a good amount of iron, but it also increases absorption of iron from other food sources.
- Don't drink a lot of tea, as it contains tannins, substances that can inhibit iron absorption. (Herbal tea is okay, though.)
- Take an iron supplement if your doctor recommends this. While iron is best absorbed when taken on an empty stomach, it can upset your stomach. Taking iron with meals is less upsetting to the stomach. *(Note: Recent research is suggesting that high levels of iron in the blood may increase the risk of heart attacks. Check with your doctor before taking iron supplements.)*
- Avoid antacids, phosphates (which are found in soft drinks, beer, ice cream, etc.) and the food additive EDTA. These block iron absorption.

CHEST PAIN

Chest pain can result from a lot of things, including:
- Heart attack
- Lung problems such as pneumonia, bronchitis, collapsed lung or a blood clot in the lung (pulmonary embolism)
- Hiatus hernia
- Heartburn
- Shingles
- Pulled muscle

- Anxiety
- Swallowing too much air

How do you know when you need medical help for chest pain? It's not always easy to tell. If you're not sure why your chest hurts, it's best to check it out. Getting help for a heart attack or lung problem could save your life.

Questions to Ask

Do you have any of these problems along with the chest pain:
- Crushing pain that spreads to the arm, neck or jaw
- Shortness of breath or trouble breathing
- Nausea and/or vomiting
- Sweating
- Uneven pulse or heartbeat
- Sense of foreboding

YES

NO

Did the chest pain arise because you were badly injured? Does it hurt all the time and/or is it getting worse?

YES

NO

flowchart continued in next column

Do you have a history of heart problems or angina? Has your prescribed medicine stopped working?

YES

NO

Have you had an operation or illness that has kept you in bed recently?

YES

NO

Do you have any of these problems as well as the chest pain?:
- Fever
- Coughing up green, yellow or blood-stained phlegm
- Shortness of breath
- Pain in the chest that is worse when breathing deeply

YES

NO

Do you have either of the following?
- Pain in the chest when you move about
- Tenderness in the muscles of the chest wall

YES

NO

flowchart continued on next page

Do you have belching and/or burning just above your stomach? Does it come and go. Does it get worse when you bend or sit down? Does the chest pain improve if you take antacids.

YES

NO

Is the chest pain only on one side and does it stay the same when you breathe?/ And do you have a burning feeling and a skin rash in the same place as the chest pain?

YES

NO

Do you have any of these problems with the chest pain:
- Palpitations
- Light-headedness
- Dizziness, feeling faint
- Pins and needles in the hands, feet and face
- Fatigue
- Anxiety

YES

NO

Has the chest pain lasted longer than two days?

YES

NO

Self-Care Procedures

After your doctor has diagnosed the cause of your chest pain, you may be able to speed your recovery by following appropriate Self-Care Procedures.

For a pulled muscle or small injury to your ribs:
- Don't strain the muscle or ribs when they hurt.
- Rest.
- Take aspirin, paracetamol or ibuprofen for the pain. *Note: Do not give aspirin, or any medication containing salicylates, to children under 12 years of age, unless directed by a doctor, due to its association with Reye's syndrome, a potentially fatal condition.*
- Call your doctor if the pain lasts more than two days.

For a hiatus hernia (a condition in which part of your stomach pushes up through your diaphragm):
- Lose weight if you are overweight.
- Eat five or six small meals a day instead of three large ones.
- Avoid tobacco, alcohol, coffee, spicy foods, peppermint, chocolate, citrus juices and fizzy drinks.
- Take antacids when you have heartburn and before you go to bed.
- Don't eat food or drink milk in the two hours before going to bed.
- Don't bend over or lie down after eating.
- Don't wear tight clothes, tight belts or corsets.
- Raise the head of your bed by 7.5 to 10 cm (3 to 4 in).

For anxiety and hyperventilation:
Some people hyperventilate (over-breathe) when they are anxious. This causes changes in the body's chemistry. As a result, nerves and muscles can be affected, causing pins and needles, palpitations and sometimes chest pain.
If you are prone to hyperventilate:

- Try to stay away from people and things that upset you.
- Talk about your anxiety with family, friends or clergy. (You may want to see a counsellor or psychiatrist if this doesn't help.)
- Don't take too much aspirin or other drugs that contain salicylates.
- Cover your mouth and nose loosely with a paper bag if you are hyperventilating. Breathe in and out at least 10 times. Take the bag away and try breathing normally. Repeat breathing in and out of the bag if you need to.

FAINTING

Just before fainting, you may feel a sense of dread followed by the sense that everything around you is swaying. You may see spots before your eyes. Then you go into a cold sweat, your face turns pale, and you topple over.

A common cause of fainting is a sudden reduction of blood flow to the brain which results from a temporary drop in blood pressure and pulse rate. These lead to a brief loss of consciousness. A fainting victim may pass out for several seconds or for a couple of minutes.

People faint for many reasons. Medical reasons include:

- Low blood sugar (hypoglycaemia), which is common in early pregnancy
- Anaemia
- Any condition in which there is a rapid loss of blood. This can be due to internal bleeding, such as from a peptic ulcer or a tubal pregnancy or burst ovarian cyst in females.
- Heart and circulatory problems such as abnormal heart rhythm, heart attack or stroke
- Eating disorders such as anorexia or bulimia

Other situations that can lead to feeling faint or fainting include:

- Extreme pain
- A sudden change in body position, such as standing up too quickly (postural hypotension)
- Sudden emotional stress or fright
- Taking some prescription medications (e.g., some of the medicines that lower high blood pressure, tranquillizers, antidepressants and even some nonprescription medicines when taken in excessive amounts)
- In women, any procedure that stretches the cervix, such as having an IUD inserted, especially in women who have never been pregnant.

Know, also, that the risk of fainting increases if you are in hot, humid weather, are in a stuffy room or have consumed excessive amounts of alcohol.

Here are some do's and don'ts to remember if someone faints:

Do's:

- Catch the person before he or she falls.
- Place the person in a horizontal position with the head below the level of the heart and the legs raised to promote blood flow to the brain. If a potential fainting victim can lie down right away, he or she may not lose consciousness.
- Turn the victim's head to the side so the tongue doesn't fall back into the throat.
- Loosen any tight clothing.
- Apply moist towels to the person's face and neck.
- If the surroundings are cold, keep the victim warm. If they are hot, keep the victim cool.

Don'ts:

- Don't slap or shake anyone who's just fainted.
- Don't try to give the person anything to eat or drink, not even water, until he or she is fully conscious.
- Don't allow the person who's fainted to get up until the sense of physical weakness passes and then be watchful for a few minutes to be sure he or she doesn't faint again.

Questions to Ask

Is the person who fainted not breathing and does he or she not have a pulse? **YES**

NO

flowchart continues in next column

Are signs of a heart attack also present with the fainting:
- Chest pain or pressure
- Pain that spreads to the arm, neck or jaw
- Shortness of breath or difficulty breathing
- Nausea and/or vomiting
- Sweating
- Rapid, slow or irregular heartbeat
- Anxiety

YES

NO

Are signs of a stroke also present with the fainting:
- Numbness or weakness in the face, arm or leg
- Temporary loss of vision or speech, double vision
- Sudden, severe headache

YES

NO

Did the fainting occur after an injury to the head? **YES**

NO

Do you have any of these with the fainting:
- Pelvic pain
- Black stools

YES

NO

Have you fainted more than once? **YES**

NO

flowchart continues on next page

Are you taking high blood pressure medication or have you recently taken a new or increased dose of prescription medicine? **YES**

NO

Self-Care Procedures

If you are feeling faint, do one of the following:
• Lie down and raise both legs.
• Sit down, bend forward and put your head between your knees.

If you faint easily:
• Get up slowly from your bed or from a sitting position.
• Follow your doctor's advice to treat any medical condition that may lead to fainting. Take medicines as prescribed, but let your doctor know about any side effects so he or she can monitor your condition.
• Don't wear tight-fitting clothing around your neck.
• Avoid turning your head suddenly.
• Try to stay out of stuffy rooms and hot, humid places. If you can't, use a fan.
• Avoid activities that can put your life in danger if you have frequent fainting spells (e.g., driving and climbing high places).
• Drink alcohol only in moderation.

For women who are pregnant:
• Get out of bed slowly.
• Keep plain biscuits at your bedside and eat a few before getting out of bed. Try other foods such as dry toast or bananas.
• Eat small, frequent meals instead of a few large ones. Include a good source of protein (e.g., lean meat, low-fat cheese and milk) in each meal. Avoid sweets. Don't skip meals or go a long time without eating.
• Don't sit for long periods of time.
• Keep your legs raised when you sit.
• When you stand, for example when in a queue, don't stand still. Move your legs to pump blood up to your heart.
• Take vitamin supplements if your doctor prescribes them.
• Never lie on your back during the last three months of pregnancy. It is best to lie on your left side. If you can't, lie on your right side.

FATIGUE

Fatigue is feeling tired, drained of energy and exhausted. Fatigue makes it hard for you to do normal daily activities. There are many causes of fatigue, both physical and emotional. Usually the cause is not serious and the problem is easily treated. In a few cases the cause is a serious disorder that needs medical attention.

Possible physical causes of fatigue include:
• Lack of sleep
• Prolonged effects of flu or a bad cold
• PMS (See page 154.)
• 'Crash dieting' or poor eating, which result in vitamin and mineral deficiencies

- Migraine headaches
- Side effects from allergies or chemical sensitivities
- Living or working in hot, humid conditions

Possible emotional effects include:
- Burnout (wearing yourself out by doing too much)
- Boredom
- Change (getting divorced, retiring from work, facing a big decision)
- Depression and/or anxiety

Possible serious underlying diseases that may cause fatigue include:
- Chronic fatigue syndrome (ME)
- Lupus (the systemic type)
- AIDS
- Tuberculosis
- Alcohol or drug abuse
- Leukaemia
- Underactive thyroid gland (hypothyroidism)

Treatment

The first thing to do is find the cause(s) of the fatigue so you know what to treat. It is important to keep track of any other symptoms that accompany the fatigue, so that both physical and emotional causes can be identified and dealt with. For example, iron supplements can help with the fatigue that results from iron-deficiency anaemia.

Questions to Ask

Do any of these problems occur with the fatigue:
- Chest pain or tightness
- Shortness of breath
- Loss of balance or weakness, especially in one part or one side of the body
- Thoughts of suicide

YES

 NO

Is the fatigue accompanied by any of these problems:
- Loss of weight of more than 3 Kg (6.6 lb) without dieting
- Yellow skin and/or eyes
- Blurry or double vision
- Excessive vomiting
- Feeling anxious, and not being able to calm down

YES

 NO

Do you have two or more of these problems with the fatigue:
- Swollen lymph glands
- Sore throat
- Headache
- Painful swelling in the neck, armpit or groin
- Fever
- Night sweats
- Excessive thirst or urination

YES

 NO

flowchart continued on next page

Do you have or have you had any of these problems:

- Arthritis or rheumatism for more than three months
- Fingers that get pale, numb or uncomfortable in the cold
- Mouth sores for more than two weeks
- Low blood counts from anaemia, low white cell count or low platelet count
- A rash on your cheeks for more than a month
- Skin rash after being in the sun
- Pain for more than two days when taking deep breaths
- Fainting episode
- Seizure, convulsion or fit

YES

NO

Did you start to feel tired or 'blue' after taking medicine?

YES

NO

Have you felt tired for more than two weeks? Are you too tired to live your normal life, and you don't know why?

YES

NO

flowchart continued in next column

For women: Are you starting menopause? Or could you be pregnant?

YES

NO

Self-Care Procedures

Eat better. Eating too much and 'crash dieting' are both hard on your body. Don't skip breakfast. Stay away from rich, sugary snacks. Eat lots of food with iron, whole-grain breads and cereals, and raw fruits and vegetables.

Get more exercise. Exercise can give you more energy and it can calm you, too. Try taking a walk in the open air if you feel tired. It can help.

Cool off. Working or playing in hot weather can sap you of energy. Living or working in a warm place without fresh air is bad, too. Rest in a cool, dry place as often as you can. Drink lots of water. Open a window when you can.

Rest and relax. A good night's sleep can make you feel much better. But you can relax during the day, too. Take breaks during your work day. Practice deep breathing or meditation.

Change your routine. Try to do something new and interesting every day. If you already do too much, make time for some peace and quiet.

FEVER

A body temperature of 37°C (98.6°F) is average. Many healthy people have temperatures a degree above or below average.

Body temperature goes up and down during the day, too. Your temperature is usually lower in the morning and higher in the evening. You may think you have a fever when you don't, particularly if you drink something hot before taking your temperature.

You can take your temperature by mouth, under the arm or with a special thermometer that you put in your ear. Skin temperature strips which you hold on the forehead do not measure temperature accurately but can give you an idea if your temperature is raised.

Here are some things that can change your body temperature:
- Wearing too many clothes
- Exercise
- Hot, humid weather
- Hormones (The hormones in a woman's body make her temperature go up a little at certain times of the month.)
- If none of these things are true and your temperature is over 37.5°C (100°F), you have a fever. Adults probably don't need to do anything if they don't feel ill. Be sure to see your doctor if you don't feel well or if the fever goes over 39.5°C (103°F).

Questions to Ask

Do any of these problems accompany the fever:
- Seizure or fit
- Listlessness
- Abnormal breathing
- Stiff neck
- Irritability
- Confusion

YES

NO

Is the person with the fever a baby younger than six months old?

YES

NO

In a child or adult: Does the person have any of these problems as well as the fever:
- Ear pain
- Persistent sore throat
- Vomiting
- Diarrhoea
- Pain or burning sensation when passing urine
- Frequent urination
- Cough with green or yellow phlegm

YES

NO

In an adult: Is the fever higher than 39.5°C (103°F)? Has it lasted more than four days even though you have tried to bring it down?

YES

NO

flowchart continued on next page

In a child: Is the fever over 38.5°C (101°F). Has it been this high for 48 hours even if you have tried to bring it down?

YES

NO

Is the fever sufferer a baby younger than 6 months of age?

YES

NO

Has the person had an operation recently? Or does the person have a long-term illness such as:
• Heart disease
• Lung disease
• Kidney disease
• Cancer
• Diabetes

YES

NO

Has the fever done any of the following:
• Gone away for more than 24 hours and then returned
• Developed soon after a visit to a foreign country

YES

NO

Self-Care Procedures

• Drink fruit squash, water and other soft drinks.

• Take a bath with warm not hot water.
• Take aspirin or paracetamol.
  Note: Do not give aspirin, or any medication containing salicylates, to children under 12 years of age, unless directed by a doctor, due to its association with Reye's syndrome, a potentially fatal condition.
• Rest in bed.
• Don't wear too many clothes or blankets.
• Don't exercise.

HEADACHES

Headaches are one of the most common health problems. They have many different causes. Most headaches do not last long and are related to stress, but sometimes a headache has a serious cause. You need to know how to recognize a headache that might need medical attention.

Kinds of Headaches

Tension, or muscular, headaches – Most people get this kind of headache. You feel a dull ache in your forehead, above your ears or at the back of your head. You get a tension headache when the muscles in your face, neck or head get tight. This can happen when you:
• Don't get enough sleep
• Are stressed
• Read for too long particularly in poor light
• Do boring work

Migraine headaches – Migraine headaches happen when blood vessels in your head close too tight and then open too wide. Women are more prone to migraines than men, and people in the same family often get them. A migraine headache makes your head throb and feels like someone is hitting it with a big hammer. Many people also get these symptoms:
- One side of the head hurts more than the other
- Nausea or vomiting
- Visual problems such as seeing spots
- Light hurts the eyes.
- Loud noises hurting the ears

Sinus headaches – Your sinuses are behind your cheeks, around your eyes, and in your nose. You get a sinus headache when your sinuses swell up. Anyone is a candidate for sinus headaches; however, people with allergies like hay fever often get them.

A sinus headache makes your forehead, cheekbones and nose hurt. It hurts more if you bend over or touch your face. You can get a sinus headache from:
- A cold
- Allergies

Headaches can also result from:
- A sensitivity to certain foods and drinks
- Alcohol
- Cigarette smoke
- Exposure to chemicals and/or pollution
- Side effects from some medications

A headache can be a symptom of many medical conditions, too. Some of these are:

- Fever
- Dental problems
- Allergies
- Depression
- High blood pressure

Less often, a headache can be a symptom of a serious health problem that needs immediate medical attention. Examples are:
- Eye problems, such as acute glaucoma
- Stroke
- Tumour, blood clot or a ruptured blood vessel (aneurysm) in the brain

How to Avoid Headaches

- Keep track of when, where and why you get headaches. If you find out what triggers a headache, try to stay away from it.
- Note early symptoms and try to abort a headache in its earliest stages (e.g., take a painkiller such as paracetamol).
- Exercise at least two or three times a week. This helps keep headaches away.
- Avoid foods and drinks that give you a headache.

Foods That Can Cause Headaches

These foods give some people headaches:
- Alcoholic drinks, especially red wine
- Aspartame (an artificial sweetener)
- Bananas
- Coffee, tea, cola and other drinks with caffeine

- Chocolate
- Grapefruits, oranges and other citrus fruits
- Food additives such as monosodium glutamate (MSG)
- Hard cheeses such as mature cheddar
- Nuts
- Onions
- Sour cream
- Vinegar

Questions to Ask

Is the headache associated with any of the following:
- A serious head injury
- A blow to the head that causes severe pain, vomiting, confusion or lethargy
- Loss of consciousness

YES

NO

Is the headache associated with any of the following:
- Pain in one eye
- Blurred vision
- Double vision
- Slurring of speech
- Confusion
- Personality change
- A problem moving the arms or legs

YES

NO

flowchart continued in next column

Is the headache associated with fever, drowsiness, nausea, vomiting or a stiff neck?

YES

NO

Has the headache been occurring for more than two to three days and increased in frequency and intensity?

YES

NO

Has the headache come on suddenly, and does it hurt more than others you have had?

YES

NO

Has the headache occurred at the same time of day, week or month?

YES

NO

Have you noticed the headache only taking newly prescribed or over-the-counter medicines?

YES

NO

Self-Care Procedures

When you have a headache:
- Rest in a dark, quiet room with your eyes closed.

- Take a hot bath.
- Put a cold facecloth over your eyes.
- Take aspirin, paracetamol or ibuprofen right away. Painkillers work best when the headache starts. *Note: Do not give aspirin, or any medication containing salicylates, to children under 12 years of age, unless directed by a doctor, due to its association with Reye's syndrome, a potentially fatal condition.*
- Relax. Try thinking of a calm, happy place. Breathe slowly and deeply.

INSOMNIA

Do you ever find yourself wide awake long after you go to bed at night? Well, you're not alone. Insomnia is extremely common. Insomniacs may find it difficult to fall asleep at night, may wake up in the middle of the night, or may wake up too early and be unable to get back to sleep. And when they're not asleep, they worry about whether or not they'll be able to sleep. They are also irritable and feel fatigued during the day.

An occasional sleepless night is nothing to worry about. But, if insomnia bothers you for three weeks or longer, it can be a real medical problem. Some medical problems that lead to insomnia include:
- Over-active thyroid gland
- Heart or lung conditions that cause shortness of breath when lying down
- Depression and anxiety disorders
- Allergies and early-morning wheezing
- Any illness, injury or surgery that causes pain and/or discomfort (e.g., arthritis) which interrupts sleep
- Sexual problems (e.g., impotence)
- Hot flushes that interrupt sleep
- Any disorder (urinary, gastrointestinal or neurological) that makes it necessary to urinate or open the bowels during the night
- Side effects of certain medications (e.g., decongestants and cortisone drugs)
  Other factors that can lead to insomnia:
- Emotional stress
- Too much noise when trying to fall asleep. This includes a snoring partner.
- The use of stimulants such as caffeine from coffee, tea or colas
- A lack of physical exercise
- Lack of a sex partner

Questions to Ask

Do you have trouble falling or staying asleep because of any of the following:
- Pain or discomfort due to illness or injury
- Waking up to go to the toilet

YES

NO

Has your sleep been disturbed since you began taking medication of any kind?

YES

NO

flowchart continued on next page

Do you still have trouble sleeping after three weeks, with or without using the Self-Care Procedures listed?

YES

NO

Self-Care Procedures

Many old-fashioned remedies for sleeplessness work for some people. Next time you find yourself unable to sleep, try these time-tested cures.

- Avoid caffeine in all forms after lunchtime. Coffee, tea, chocolate, colas and some other soft drinks contain this stimulant, as do certain over-the-counter and prescription drugs. Check the labels for content.

- Avoid naps during the day. Naps decrease the quality of night-time sleep.

- Avoid more than one or two alcoholic drinks at dinnertime and during the rest of the evening. Even though alcohol is a sedative, it can disrupt sleep. Always check with your doctor about alcohol consumption if you are taking medications.

- A hot milky drink and a plain biscuit at bedtime may help you get to sleep.

- Take a long, warm bath before bedtime. This soothes and unwinds tense muscles, leaving you relaxed enough to fall asleep.

- Read a book or perform a repetitive activity such as needlework. Try not to

watch TV or listen to the radio. These kinds of distractions may hold your attention and keep you awake.

- Make your bedroom as comfortable as possible. Create a quiet, dark atmosphere. Use clean, fresh sheets and pillows, and keep the room temperature comfortable (neither too warm nor too cool).

- Ban worry from the bedroom. Don't allow yourself to go over the mistakes of the day in your mind as you toss and turn. You're off duty now. The idea is to associate your bed with sleep.

- Develop a regular bedtime routine. Locking or checking doors and windows, brushing your teeth and reading before you turn in every night prepare you for sleep.

- Count those sheep! Counting slowly is a soothing, hypnotic activity. By picturing repetitive, monotonous images, you may bore yourself to sleep.

- Try listening to recordings made especially to help promote sleep. Check local bookshops.

- Don't take over-the-counter sleeping pills for longer than two or three days without your doctor's permission.

REPETITIVE STRAIN INJURIES

Repetitive strain injuries (RSIs) can occur when you perform the same activity over and over for a long period of time either at work, at home, during sports and/or hobbies. The types of movements involved include repeated forceful:

- Drilling or hammering
- Lifting
- Pushing or pulling
- Squeezing, twisting
- Wrist, finger and hand movements

Symptoms of RSI include generalized pain in the wrist and hand, initially occurring only during or after the activity but eventually becoming continuous even at rest. Some people with these symptoms will be found to have tendinitis, carpal tunnel syndrome (CTS) or localized inflammation where muscles attach to bone (e.g.. in tennis elbow).

Typical problems that result from RSIs are:

Tendinitis – Constant wear and tear on wrists, elbows and shoulders may create tiny tears in the tendons, causing swelling, inflammation and pain. Tendinitis tends to hurt more at night than during the day. Treatment for tendinitis varies with the cause and how severe it is.

Carpal Tunnel Syndrome (CTS) – Develops when tissues swell inside the carpal tunnel, a narrow tunnel in the wrist. Soft tissue in this tunnel enlarges, pinching the nerve that passes through it. Women are more likely to suffer from CTS than men because their carpal tunnel is usually smaller. Pregnancy can also increase a woman's risk of CTS, though the pain usually disappears after the baby is born.

CTS is easier to treat and less likely to cause future problems if it is diagnosed early. See 'Preventing Wrist and Hand Injuries' on page 96. Once diagnosed,

CTS can be treated with:
- Physiotherapy
- Wearing a splint at night
- Taking anti-inflammatory medicines such as aspirin or ibuprofen
- Changing the workplace set-up to reduce pressure in the wrist

Sometimes surgery is necessary if these measures aren't enough.

Repetitive strain injuries are on the increase. In many cases, computers are the culprits. A writer or a busy secretary, for example, often strikes the keys about 200,000 times a day; that's like your fingers taking a 10-mile walk. And chairs without lumbar support can cause back pain. Misplaced monitors can bring on eyestrain and stiff necks. No wonder many keyboard operators experience tendinitis and CTS.

Questions to Ask

Do you have chest pain and any of these problems:
- Pain that spreads to the arm, neck or jaw
- Pressure, especially on the left side
- Shortness of breath or trouble breathing
- Uneven pulse or heartbeat
- Nausea and/or vomiting
- Sweating
- Feeling anxious or light headed

YES

 NO

flowchart continued on next page

95

Do you have:
- Severe or persistent pain, swelling or spasm
- Tenderness or stiffness and limited motion in the affected area such as the shoulder, arm or wrist

YES

NO

Does pain in your hand, shoulder or wherever wake you from sleep?

YES

NO

Have you:
- Suffered pain, numbness and tingling in your hand for more than two weeks
- Been unable to make a fist for a couple of weeks

YES

NO

Do you frequently drop object(s) and does your thumb feel weak?

YES

NO

Self-Care and Preventive Procedures

For preventing wrist and hand injuries:

Whenever your hands and wrists perform the same activity time and again, you increase your risk of CTS and tendinitis. Change how you do a task and you may avoid some of these injuries.

- Keep your wrists straight when typing. Make sure your fingers are lower than your wrists and don't rest the heels of your hands on the keyboard. Try a wrist rest for your keyboard to keep your wrists higher than the keyboard. Drop and tip your keyboard or try one of the new ergonomic keyboards.
- Do not hold an object in the same position for a long time. Even simple tasks such as hammering a nail can cause injury when performed over a period of time.
- Give your hands a break by resting them for a few minutes each hour.
- Lift objects with your whole hand or, better yet, with both hands. Gripping or lifting with the thumb and index finger puts stress on your wrist.
- If your kind of work causes pain in your hands and wrists, see if you can share different jobs with someone else. Or alternate the stressful tasks with other work.
  - Exercise your hands and wrists as often as possible.
  - Stretch your hands. Place them in front, spread your fingers as far apart as possible and hold for five seconds. Relax. Repeat five times with each hand.
  - Turn your wrists in a circle, palms up and then palms down. Relax your fingers and keep your elbows still. Repeat five times.
  - Drop your hands downwards. Shake your hands up and down, then sideways, until the tension is gone.

For carpal tunnel syndrome:

- Lose weight. CTS is linked to obesity; the excess tissue can press on the carpal tunnel.
- Take aspirin or ibuprofen if you can tolerate it, to reduce the pain and inflammation. *Note: Do not give aspirin, or any medication containing salicylates, to children under 12 years of age, unless directed by a doctor, due to its association with Reye's syndrome, a potentially fatal condition.*

For preventing tendinitis:

- Use proper posture, proper equipment and proper technique when doing repetitive tasks.
- Take stretch breaks several times a day.
- Do stretching and strengthening exercises to keep your shoulder, neck and arm muscles strong and flexible. See also: 'Treating Tendinitis' on p. 74.

SNORING

Snoring is the sound made when the upper airway is blocked during sleep. It can result from a number of things, including obesity, enlarged tonsils and adenoids, and deformities in the nasal passages. Smoking, heavy drinking, overeating (especially before bedtime) and allergies can lead to snoring by causing the nasal passages to swell and blocking the free flow of air. Also, people who sleep on their backs are more likely to snore because the tongue falls back towards the throat and partly closes the airway. Nine out of 10 snorers are men, and most of them are age 40 or older.

Snoring can be merely a nuisance or can be a signal of a serious health problem, sleep apnoea, which may need treatment. In sleep apnoea breathing stops for at least 10 seconds, but usually for 20 to 30 seconds or even up to one or two minutes during sleep. It is more common in men than in women and typically affects men who are middle-aged and older. It can result from:

- An obstructed airway. This is more common as people age, especially in those who are obese or who have smoked for many years.
- Rarely, a central nervous system disorder such as a stroke or a brain tumour
- A chronic respiratory disease or a respiratory allergy such as rhinitis

Questions to Ask

Do you notice the following signs of sleep apnoea during your daytime hours:

- Sleepiness or chronic daytime drowsiness
- Poor memory and concentration
- Irritability
- Falling asleep while driving or working
- Loss of sex drive
- Headaches particularly on waking

YES

NO

flowchart continued on next page

Has your partner ever noticed that your breathing has stopped for 10 seconds or longer while you are snoring? **YES**

NO

Has snoring persisted despite using the Self-Care Procedures listed? **YES**

NO

Self-Care Procedures

• Sleep on your side. Prop an extra pillow behind your back so you won't roll over. Try sleeping on a narrow sofa for a few nights to get accustomed to staying on your side.

• Sew a large marble or tennis ball into a pocket on the back of your pyjamas. The discomfort it causes will remind you to sleep on your side.

• If you must sleep on your back, raise the head of the bed by putting bricks or blocks between the mattress and box spring. Or buy a wedge especially made to be placed between the mattress and box spring to elevate the head section. Elevating the head prevents the tongue from falling against the back of the throat.

• If you are heavy, lose weight. Excess fatty tissue in the throat can cause snoring.

• Don't drink alcohol or eat a heavy meal in the three hours before bedtime. For some reason, both seem to foster snoring.

• If necessary, take an antihistamine or decongestant before retiring to relieve nasal congestion (which can also contribute to snoring). *(Note: Older men should check with their doctors before taking decongestants. Decongestants containing ephedrine can cause urinary problems in older men.)*

• Get rid of allergens in the bedroom such as dust, down-filled (feather) pillows and duvets. This may also relieve nasal congestion.

• Try over-the-counter 'nasal strips'. These keep the nostrils open and lift them up, keeping nasal passages unobstructed.

URINARY INCONTINENCE

If you have urinary incontinence, you suffer from a loss of bladder control or your body fails to store urine properly. As a result, you can't prevent yourself from passing urine, even though you may try to hold it in. Urinary incontinence is not a normal part of ageing, but often affects older people because the sphincter muscles that open the bladder into the urethra become less efficient with ageing.

Although you might feel embarrassed if you have urinary incontinence, you should nevertheless let your doctor know about it. It could be a symptom of a disorder that could lead to more trouble if not treated and, in most cases, the problem is treatable.

Two categories of urinary incontinence are acute incontinence and persistent incontinence.

The acute form is generally a symptom of a new illness or condition (e.g., bladder infection, inflammation of the prostate, urethra or vagina, or constipation).

Side effects of some medications such as diuretics (water pills), tranquillizers and antihistamines can also result in acute urinary incontinence.

Acute urinary incontinence comes on suddenly. It is often easily reversed when the condition that caused it is treated.

Persistent incontinence comes on gradually over time. It lingers or remains, even after other conditions or illnesses have been treated. There are many types of persistent incontinence. The three types that account for 80 per cent of cases are:

Stress Incontinence – Urine leaks out when there is a sudden rise in pressure in the abdomen. The amount ranges from small leaks to large spills. Stress incontinence typically happens when coughing, sneezing, laughing, lifting, jumping or running or when straining to open the bowels. Stress incontinence is more common in women than in men.

Urge Incontinence – This is an inability to control the bladder when the urge to urinate occurs comes on suddenly, so there is often not enough time to make it to the toilet. This type typically results in large accidents. It can be caused by a number of things, including an enlarged prostate gland, a spinal cord injury, multiple sclerosis or Parkinson's disease.

Mixed Incontinence – This type has elements of both stress and urge incontinence.

Other types of persistent incontinence are:

Overflow Incontinence – Constant dribbling of urine occurs because the bladder is overfull. This may be due to an enlarged prostate, diabetes or multiple sclerosis.

Functional Incontinence – With this, a person has trouble getting to the toilet quickly enough, even though he or she has bladder control. This can happen in a person who is physically disabled.

Total Incontinence – In this rare type, with complete loss of bladder control, urine leakage can be continual. It may result from a structural problem, such as an opening between the bladder and the vagina.

Care and treatment for urinary incontinence will depend on the type and cause(s). The first step is to find out if there is an underlying problem and then attempt to correct it. Treatment can also include pelvic floor exercises and other Self-Care Procedures, along with medication, collagen injections into the neck of the bladder (for a certain type of stress incontinence) or surgery to correct the specific problem.

Your GP may evaluate and treat your incontinence or send you to a urologist, a doctor who specializes in treating problems of the bladder and urinary tract.

Questions to Ask

Have you lost control of your bladder after an injury to your spine or back? **YES**

NO

Does your loss of bladder control come with any of these symptoms:
- Loss of consciousness
- Inability to speak or slurred speech
- Loss of sight, double or blurred vision
- Sudden, severe headaches
- Paralysis, weakness or loss of sensation in an arm, or leg and/or the face on the same side of the body
- Change in personality, behaviour and/or emotions
- Confusion and dizziness

YES

NO

Is the loss of bladder control more than temporary after surgery or an abdominal injury? **YES**

NO

flowchart continued in next column

Do you have any of these problems with loss of bladder control:
- Fever and chills
- Back pain (sometimes severe) in one or both sides of the lower back or just about your midline
- Frequent urination accompanied by a burning sensation
- Blood in the urine or cloudy urine
- Abdominal pain
- Nausea or vomiting

YES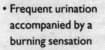

NO

With the loss of bladder control, do you have diabetes or symptoms of diabetes such as:
- Extreme thirst
- Unusual hunger
- Excessive loss or gain in weight
- Blurred vision
- Easy fatigue, drowsiness
- Slow healing of cuts and/or skin infections

YES

NO

flowchart continued on next page

If you are a man, do you:
- Dribble urine and/or feel the need to urinate again after you have finished urinating
- Pass small amounts of urine many times during the day
- Often wake to urinate at night
- Often have an intense and sudden need to urinate
- Have a slow, weak or interrupted stream of urine

YES

NO

Do you leak urine when you cough, sneeze, laugh, jump, run or lift heavy objects?

YES

NO

Did you lose some bladder control only after taking a new medicine or after taking a higher dose of a medicine you were already taking?

YES

NO

Self-Care Procedures

- Do exercises to strengthen your pelvic floor muscles. They can help treat or

cure stress incontinence. Even elderly women who have leaked urine for years can benefit greatly from these exercises. Here's how to do them:
- First, identify where your pelvic floor muscles are. One way to do this is to start to urinate, then hold back and try to stop. If you can slow the stream of urine, even a little, you are using the right muscles. You should feel muscles squeezing around your urethra and anus.
- Next, relax your body, close your eyes and just imagine that you are going to urinate and then hold back from doing so. You should feel the muscles squeeze like you did in the step before this one.
- Squeeze the muscles for three seconds and then relax them for three seconds. When you squeeze and relax, count slowly. Start by doing this three times a day. Gradually work up to three sets of 10 contractions, holding each one for 10 seconds at a time. You can do them in lying, sitting and/or standing positions. As no one can tell that you are doing the exercises, you can do them in spare moments such as while waiting for a bus.
- When you do these exercises:
  - Do not tense the muscles in your abdomen or buttocks.
  - Do not hold your breath, clench your fists or teeth or make a face.
  - If you are not sure you're doing the exercise correctly, consult your doctor.
- Squeeze your pelvic floor muscles just before and during whatever it is (coughing, sneezing, jumping, etc.) that

causes you to lose urine. Relax the muscles once the activity is over.
- It may take several months to benefit from pelvic floor exercises and you need to keep doing them daily to maintain their benefit.

Other Self-Care Procedures

- Avoid or limit drinks containing caffeine (e.g., coffee, tea, colas, chocolate).
- Limit carbonated drinks, alcohol, citrus juices, greasy and spicy foods and items containing artificial sweeteners. These can irritate the bladder.
- Drink 1 to 2 litres (1 1/2 to 3 pints) of water throughout the day.
- Go to the toilet often, even if you don't feel the urge. When you urinate, empty your bladder as much as you can. Relax for a minute or two and then try to go again. Keep a diary of when you have episodes of incontinence. If you find that you have accidents every three hours, for example, empty your bladder every 2 1/2 hours. Use an alarm clock or wristwatch with an alarm to remind you.
- Wear clothes you can remove quickly and easily when you use the toilet. Examples are clothes with elasticated waists or with velcro closures or press fasteners instead of buttons and zips. Also, look for belts that are easy to undo or don't wear belts at all.
- Wear absorbent pads or briefs.

To reduce the chances of accidents:
- Empty your bladder before you leave the house, take a nap or go to bed.
- Keep the pathway to your toilet free of clutter and well lit. Make sure the toilet door is left open until you use it.
- Use an elevated toilet seat and have a rail fitted if these will make it easier for you to get on and off the toilet.
- Consider keeping a bedpan, plastic urinal (for men) or portable commode chair near your bed. You can get these at pharmacies or medical supply shops.

URINARY TRACT INFECTIONS (UTIs)

About one out of five women will get a urinary tract infection (UTI) during the course of her lifetime. Some women get many UTIs. Men get UTIs, too, but not as often as women do.

What is the urinary tract? Your urinary tract is made up of these parts:
- Kidneys
- Bladder
- Ureters (tubes that connect the kidneys to the bladder)
- Urethra (the tube through which urine leaves the body)

How do we get UTIs? Usually, bacteria enter through the urethra and travel to the bladder. They grow in the bladder and can also migrate to the ureters and kidneys.

Bacteria can get into a woman's urethra during sex. You should go to the bathroom right after sex to flush the bacteria out. Women who use a diaphragm for birth control have twice the risk of getting a UTI. Changes that happen during pregnancy and after the menopause can also make a woman prone to UTIs.

Also, irritation to the opening of the urethra can lead to inflammation of the bladder (cystitis). If you have signs of a vaginal infection (discharge, foul odour, etc.), get treatment for it to help prevent a bladder infection.

Some people are born with urinary tract problems that pave the way for UTIs. Later in life, anything that keeps you from passing urine freely can lead to UTIs. Kidney stones or an enlarged prostate gland are two examples. You are also more likely to get a UTI if you have had such infections before.

Sometimes you don't even know you have a UTI. Most often you will have symptoms, though. They come suddenly, with no warning. Here are some of them:

- A strong need to go to urinate
- More frequent urination than usual
- A sharp pain or burning sensation in the urethra when you pass urine
- Blood in the urine
- Feeling like your bladder is still full after you pass urine
- Soreness in your abdomen, back, or sides
- Chills, fever, nausea

See a doctor if you have any of these symptoms. A UTI can be serious if you don't treat it. The doctor will test a sample of your urine to confirm the cause of the problem. An antibiotic to treat the infection and painkillers, if necessary, are the usual course of treatment.

How to Avoid Urinary Tract Infections

Here are some things you can do to avoid getting UTIs:

- If you're a woman, wipe from front to back after using the toilet. This keeps bacteria away from the urethra.
- Drink plenty of liquids, at least 2 to 3 litres (3 to 4½ pints) daily to flush out your body. Drink fruit juices, especially cranberry juice.
- Empty your bladder as soon as you feel the urge. Don't give bacteria a chance to grow.
- Drink a glass of water before you have sex. Urinate as soon as you can after sex, even if you don't have the urge to.
- If you use a lubricant when you have sex, use a water-soluble one like K-Y Jelly.
- Wear cotton underwear. Bacteria like a warm, wet environment. Cotton helps keep you cool and dry because it lets air flow through.
- Don't take bubble baths if you have had UTIs before. Take showers instead of baths.
- Don't wear tight jeans, trousers or underwear.
- If you use a diaphragm for birth control, clean it after each use and have it checked every year to make sure it still fits. The size may need to be changed if you gain or lose weight or if you have a

baby. Replace your diaphragm according to your doctor's advice.

Questions to Ask

Do you have any of these symptoms?
- Fever and chills
- Back pain on one or both sides of your lower back
- Vomiting and nausea

YES

NO

Do you have these problems?
- Burning sensation when you pass urine
- Passing urine a lot more often than usual
- Bloody or cloudy urine
- Pain in your abdomen or over your bladder
- Nausea or a feeling that you're going to vomit
- Fever

YES

NO

flowchart continued in next column

Do you have these problems?
- You urinate a lot, even at night
- You feel like you have an urgent need to urinate
- You feel like your bladder is still full after you urinate
- It stings when you pass urine
- It hurts to have sexual intercourse

YES

NO

Have you had symptoms for more than three days, without getting better? Did medication the doctor prescribed give you side effects (e.g., skin rash or nausea)?

YES

NO

Do you often get UTIs?

YES

NO

Self-Care Procedures

- Avoid alcohol, spicy foods and coffee.
- Drink at least 2 to 3 litres (3 to 4½ pints) of water a day. Liquids help wash out the infection.
- Get plenty of rest.

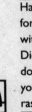

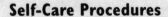

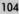

- Check for fever twice a day. Take your temperature in the morning and then in the afternoon or evening.
- Take aspirin, paracetamol or ibuprofen. *Note: Do not give aspirin, or any medication containing salicylates, to children under 12 years of age, unless directed by a doctor, due to its association with Reye's syndrome, a potentially fatal condition.*
- Go to the toilet as soon as you feel the need.
- If you feel UTI symptoms coming on, drink $^1/_2$ litre ($^3/_4$ pint) of water immediately and another $^1/_2$ litre ($^3/_4$ pint) during the next hour. This may flush out the infection and abort the attack. Over-the-counter remedies for cystitis relieve the symptoms by making the urine alkaline, but you shouldn't take them if you have a history of kidney disease.
- Empty your bladder after sex.

See your doctor if you don't feel better in three days.

CHAPTER 7
MENTAL HEALTH CONDITIONS

ALCOHOLISM

Alcoholism is the most common drug abuse problem in the UK. Abuse occurs in one of several ways: getting drunk daily, drinking a lot at certain times such as every weekend, binges of heavy drinking for weeks or months with long periods of not drinking, and infrequent drinking with loss of control over drinking.

Alcoholism is a disease which affects the alcoholic's physical health, emotional well-being and behaviour.

Physical Effects

- Impairs mental/physical reflexes
- Increases the risk of diseases such as cancer of the tongue, mouth, oesophagus, larynx, liver and bladder; cirrhosis of the liver and hepatitis; ulcers and gastritis, and irreversible brain damage when used heavily. It can also cause heart and blood pressure problems.
- Can lead to malnutrition
- Is known to cause birth defects

Emotional and Behavioural Effects

- Alters inhibitions and, therefore, may cause someone to do things he or she might not do otherwise (e.g., driving at high speeds or other daredevil acts)
- Alters mood, resulting in anger, violent behaviour, depression or even suicide — effects that can intensify as more alcohol is consumed
- May result in memory loss
- Makes family life chaotic. The divorce rate is seven times higher among alcoholics, and children of alcoholics may have long-lasting emotional problems
- Often results in decreased work attendance and performance as well as problems in dealing with employees and colleagues

Treatment

Alcoholism has a biological basis. The tendency to become alcoholic is inherited. Both men and women are four times more likely to become alcoholics if their parents were alcoholics.

Treating alcoholism as an illness is important and one thing is certain: The only way to beat a drinking problem is to stop drinking. This can be done through self-help groups such as Alcoholics

Anonymous, alcohol rehabilitation centres and psychotherapy. A prescription drug, Antabuse, is available to help in treatment. This causes violent physical reactions if a person drinks alcohol while taking the medication.

Questions to Ask

Have you had memory lapses or blackouts due to drinking? **YES**

NO

Do you continue to drink even though you have health problems caused by alcohol? **YES**

NO

Do you have to drink alcohol in order to get you through the day? **YES**

NO

Do you get withdrawal symptoms such as headaches, chills, shakes and a strong craving for alcohol and, as a result, drink more to get rid of these symptoms? **YES**

NO

flowchart continued in next column

Are you engaged in high-risk behaviour such as having unsafe sex in a non-monogamous relationship or driving a boat or car when under the influence of alcohol? Has drinking significantly affected your work, school and/or relationships with others? **YES**

NO

Do you drink to cope with stressful life events or to escape from ongoing problems? **YES**

NO

Do you tell yourself that you don't have a problem with alcohol or hide it from others and lie about your alcohol use? Or have your friends, family or employer commented about your alcohol use? **YES**

NO

Self-Care Procedures

If you are a heavy drinker, the sooner you stop drinking alcohol, the better your chances of avoiding the serious physical and psychological effects.

• Admit to your drinking. This is the first

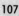

and most important step to avoid becoming an alcohol abuser.

- Change your lifestyle. Try to stay out of situations where alcohol is prominent (e.g., clubs, dances and parties) until you can control your drinking. Once you've done this, order soft drinks if you attend places where alcohol is served.
- If your friends insist you drink alcohol in order to socialize with them, make it clear that you're serious about stopping. If this is unacceptable to them, find new friends.
- Attend self-help group meetings for alcoholics, such as those organized by Alcoholics Anonymous.
- Ask your GP about any local self-help groups.
- If your employers have an Employee Assistance Programme (EAP), make use of it.

To avoid becoming alcohol dependent:

- Know your limit and stick to it.
- Drink slowly. This will help you drink less.
- Pour less alcohol and more mixer in each drink.
- Alternate an alcoholic drink with a non-alcoholic one.
- Eat while drinking. Food helps absorb alcohol in the system.
- Talk to persons who will listen to your feelings and concerns without judging you. You will be less likely to turn to alcohol to 'drown your sorrows'.
- Find ways to calm yourself other than with alcohol (e.g., hobbies, relaxation exercises, physical activities and watching films).

- Realize that you are a role model for your children. They learn from what they see. When you drink, do so responsibly.
- Don't mix drinking with driving, drugs or operating machines. These combinations can be fatal.

ANXIETY

Anxiety is a sense of dread, fear or distress over a real or imagined threat to your mental or physical well-being. Symptoms of anxiety include:

- Rapid pulse and/or breathing rate
- Racing or pounding heart
- Dry mouth
- Sweating
- Trembling
- Shortness of breath
- Faintness
- Numbness/tingling of the hands, feet or other body part
- Feeling a 'lump in the throat'
- Stomach problems

A certain amount of anxiety is normal. It can prompt you to study for a test or alert you to seek safety when you are in physical danger. Anxiety is not normal, though, when there is no apparent reason for it or when it is overwhelming and interferes with day-to-day living.

Anxiety can be a symptom of medical conditions such as:

- Heart attack
- Over-active thyroid gland

Withdrawal symptoms from nicotine, alcohol, drugs of abuse or medicines such as sleeping pills

- Low blood sugar (hypoglycaemia)
- Excess of hormones made by the adrenal glands, which are located above the kidneys
- Side effect of some medications

Anxiety can sometimes be a symptom of illnesses known as anxiety disorders. These include:

Phobias – Disorders in which terror, dread or panic results when a person is faced with a feared object, situation or activity. Examples include specific phobias (such as fear of spiders), social phobias (such as the fear of speaking in front of other people) and complex phobias (such as agoraphobia, the fear of being in places or situations from which escape might be difficult or embarrassing). Agoraphobia can occur with or without panic disorder, defined below.

Panic Attacks – Brief periods of acute anxiety that can occur without warning. Symptoms include shortness of breath, chest discomfort, heart palpitations, sweating and choking. A person having a panic attack for the first time may think he or she is having a heart attack. Panic attacks may or may not be associated with agoraphobia.

Panic disorder is thought to exist when panic attacks:
- Occur without warning
- Take place for one month, and
- Are followed by: the ongoing fear that another panic attack will occur; worry about implications of the attack or its consequences; or a significant change in behaviour

Obsessive-Compulsive Disorder – An anxiety disorder where the sufferer has persistent, involuntary thoughts or images (obsessions) and engages in ritualistic acts such as washing their hands according to certain self-imposed rules (compulsions).

Post-Traumatic Stress Disorder – A condition where a person re-experiences a traumatic past event such as a rape, war-time situation or hostage-taking. Symptoms include nightmares, flashbacks of the event, excessive alertness and emotional numbness to people and activities.

When anxiety is mild and/or does not interfere with daily living, it can be dealt with using the listed Self-Care Procedures. Professional treatment for anxiety disorders includes:
- Treatment of the medical condition, if one exists, which causes the anxiety
- Psychotherapy
- Medication

Self-help groups can also be helpful.

Questions to Ask

Do you have thoughts of suicide that don't go away? Are you planning ways to commit suicide? YES

NO

flowchart continued on next page

Are any of these problems present with the anxiety:
- Chest pain (note if it spreads, or radiates, to the arm, neck or jaw)
- Feeling of pressure, especially on the left side of the chest
- Shortness of breath or difficulty in breathing
- Nausea, vomiting, belching
- Sweating
- Irregular heartbeat

YES

NO

Are these problems present with the anxiety:
- Accumulation of fat on the neck, face and trunk
- Excessive growth of body hair
- Round face and puffy eyes
- Skin changes (e.g., reddening, thinning and stretch marks)

YES

NO

Do you have these problems with the anxiety:
- Rapid heartbeat
- Hyperactivity
- Weight loss
- Muscle weakness, tremors
- Bulging eyes
- Feeling hot or warm all the time

YES

NO

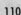

flowchart continued in next column

Does the anxiety take place only at these times:
- When you don't eat or when you physically tax yourself too much, especially if you have diabetes
- Premenstrually, for women

YES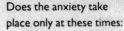

NO

Did you get the anxiety only after:
- Taking an over-the-counter (OTC) or prescription medicine
- Withdrawing from medication, nicotine, alcohol or drugs

YES

NO

Have you had any of these:
- Panic attacks followed for one month by fears of getting another one
- Worry about the implications of the attack or its consequences or
- A significant change in behaviour related to the attacks

YES

NO

flowchart continued on next page

110

If you have been through or seen a traumatic event, do you suffer from any of these problems:

- Nightmares, night terrors and/or flashbacks of the event
- Lack of concentration, poor memory, unable to sleep
- Feelings of guilt for surviving the event
- Easily startled by loud noises or anything that reminds you of the event
- Lack of interest in the activities and people you once enjoyed

YES

NO

Do any of these keep you from doing your daily activities:

- Fear of having a panic attack
- Fear of leaving the house or of being left alone
- Checking something over and over again (e.g., seeing if you've locked the door even though it is locked)
- Repeated, unwanted thoughts such as worrying you could harm someone
- Repeated, senseless acts such as washing your hands over and over again

YES

NO

Is anxiety in general keeping you from doing the things you need to do every day?

YES

NO

Self-Care Procedures

- Look for the cause of the stress that results in anxiety and deal with it directly.
- Lessen your exposure to things that cause you distress.
- Eat healthily and at regular times. Don't skip meals.
- If you develop symptoms at times when your blood sugar might be low, such as after missing a meal, eat five to six small meals per day instead of three larger ones. Carry a quick source of sugar with you at all times (e.g., dextrose tablets or sugar cubes).
- Exercise regularly.
- Avoid caffeine, nicotine and alcohol.
- Do some form of relaxation exercise daily (e.g., biofeedback, deep muscle relaxation, meditation and deep breathing exercises).
- Don't 'bite off more than you can chew'. Plan your schedule for what you can handle both physically and mentally.
- Rehearse for events that are coming up in which you have felt anxious in the past or think will cause anxiety. Several times before the event, imagine yourself feeling calm and in control as the event takes place.

flowchart continued in next column

111

- Be prepared to deal with symptoms of anxiety if you anticipate they will happen. For example, if you have hyperventilated in the past, carry a paper bag with you. If you do hyperventilate, cover your mouth and nose with the paper bag. Breathe into the paper bag slowly and rebreathe the air. Breathe in and out at least 10 times. Remove the bag and breathe normally for a few minutes. Repeat breathing in and out of the paper bag as needed.
- Help others. The positive feelings this can create can help you overcome or forget about your anxiety.

DEPRESSION

Life changes, such as divorce, death of a loved one or loss of a job can leave a person feeling depressed. So can worrying about financial problems or illness. And sometimes you may feel empty and depressed for no apparent reason. Some depression is normal and is a part of almost every person's life. Depression can, however, be a side effect of certain medicines, illnesses, or alcoholism, or be a disease in and of itself. Even the lack of natural, unfiltered sunlight between late autumn and spring can lead to a type of depression in some sensitive people. This is commonly called seasonal affective disorder (SAD).

Whatever the cause, depression can be treated. Treatment includes medicines, psychotherapy and other therapies specific to the cause of the depression, such as exposure to bright light (similar to sunlight) for depression that results from SAD.

Symptoms of depression include:
- Persistent feelings of sadness or emptiness
- Feelings of helplessness, hopelessness, guilt and worthlessness
- Loss of interest in pleasurable activities, including sex
- Sleep disturbances
- Fatigue
- Loss of energy or enthusiasm
- Difficulty in concentrating or making decisions
- Ongoing physical symptoms such as headaches or digestive disorders that don't respond to treatment
- Crying, tearfulness
- Poor appetite and weight loss, or overeating and weight gain

Questions to Ask

Have you attempted suicide? Are you planning ways to commit suicide?

flowchart continued on next page

112

Have you had markedly diminished interest or pleasure in almost all activities most of the day, nearly every day for at least two weeks? Or have you been in a depressed mood most of the day, nearly every day, and have you experienced any of the following, for at least two weeks:

- Feeling lethargic, or restless and unable to sit still
- Feeling worthless or guilty
- Changes in appetite or weight loss or gain
- Thoughts of death or suicide
- Problems in concentrating, thinking, remembering, or making decisions
- Trouble sleeping or sleeping too much
- Loss of energy or feeling tired all the time
- Headaches
- Other aches and pains
- Digestive problems
- Sexual problems
- Feelings of pessimism or hopelessness
- Anxious feelings or worry

YES

NO

flowchart continued in next column

Has depression interfered with daily activities for more than three weeks? Have you withdrawn from normal activities during this time? **YES**

NO

Has the depression appeared after taking over-the-counter or prescription medicine? **YES**

NO

Is the depression associated with dark, cloudy weather or with winter, and does it lift when spring comes? **YES**

NO

Self-Care Procedures

To overcome mild, hard-to-explain depression, try these approaches:

- Substitute a positive thought for every negative thought that pops into your head.
- Associate with congenial people, not negative people. They'll lift your morale.
- To focus your attention away from yourself, do something to help someone else.
- Get some physical exercise every day, even if it's just taking the dog for a walk. If you can do something more

113

exhilarating (e.g., biking or playing tennis), that's even better.

- Do something different. Walk or drive to somewhere new, or try a new restaurant.
- Challenge yourself with a new project. It doesn't have to be difficult, but it should be enjoyable. Do something that you enjoy and that allows you to express yourself (e.g., writing and painting).
- Do something that will make you relax. Listen to soft music, read a good book, take a warm bath or shower, do relaxation exercises.
- Talk to a friend, relative, colleague or anyone who will allow you to vent the tensions and frustrations that you are experiencing.
- Avoid drugs and alcohol. Drinking too much alcohol and the use of drugs can cause or worsen depression.
- If you find that your depression worsens or doesn't lift don't be afraid to seek professional help.

STRESS

Stress is the way our bodies react both physically and emotionally to any change in the status quo – good, bad, real or even imagined. Some physical symptoms created by stress include an increased heart rate, rapid breathing, tense muscles and increased blood pressure. Emotional reactions include irritability, anger, losing one's temper, shouting, lack of concentration and being jumpy. When left unchecked, stress may lead to a variety of health problems, including

insomnia, ulcers, back pain, colitis, high blood pressure, heart disease or reduced efficiency of the body's immune system.

Questions to Ask

Are you so distressed that you have recurrent thoughts of suicide or death? Do you have impulses or plans to commit violence? **YES**

NO

Are you experiencing frequent anxiety, nervousness, crying spells and confusion about how to handle your problems? **YES**

NO

Are you abusing alcohol, drugs (illegal or prescription) to deal with stress? **YES**

NO

flowchart continued on next page

Have you been in or involved in or witnessed a traumatic event in the past (e.g., armed combat, a plane crash, rape or assault), and do you now experience any of the following:
- Flashbacks (reliving the stressful event), painful memories, nightmares
- Feeling easily startled and/or irritable
- Feeling 'emotionally numb' and detached from others and the outside world
- Having difficulty falling asleep and/or staying asleep
- Anxiety and/or depression

YES

NO

Do you find yourself withdrawing from friends, relatives and colleagues and/or becoming angry with them at the slightest provocation?

YES

NO

Do you suffer from a medical illness that you are unable to cope with? Is this causing you not to get proper treatment?

YES

NO

Self-Care Procedures

Being able to manage stress is important in living a healthy, happy and productive life. Here are some techniques and strategies for effectively dealing with stress:
- Maintain a regular programme of healthy eating and adequate sleep.
- Exercise regularly. This promotes physical fitness as well as emotional well-being.
- Balance work and play. All work and no play can make you feel stressed. Plan some time for hobbies and recreation. These activities relax your mind and are a good respite from life's worries.
- Help others. We concentrate on ourselves when we're distressed. Sometimes helping others is the perfect remedy for whatever is troubling us.
- Take a shower or bath with warm water. This will soothe and calm your nerves and relax your muscles.
- Have a good cry or a good laugh. Both of these can make you feel better.
- Learn acceptance. Sometimes a difficult problem is out of your control. When this happens, accept it until changes can be made. This is better than worrying and getting nowhere.
- Talk out troubles. It sometimes helps to talk with a friend, relative or member of the clergy. Another person can help you see a problem from a different point of view.
- Escape for a little while. When you feel you are getting nowhere with a problem, a temporary diversion can help. Going to a movie, reading a book,

visiting a museum or taking a drive can help you get out of a rut. Temporarily leaving a difficult situation can help you develop new attitudes.

- Reward yourself. Starting today, reward yourself with little things that make you feel good. Treat yourself to a bubble bath, phone a friend, buy a flower, picnic in the park at lunchtime, try a new perfume or just give yourself some 'me' time.

- Do relaxation exercises daily. Good ones include visualization (imagining a soothing, restful scene), deep muscle relaxation (tensing and relaxing muscle fibres), meditation and deep breathing. You can learn relaxation techniques from books or tapes or at a class.

- Budget your time. Make a 'to-do list'. Rank in priority your daily tasks. Avoid committing yourself to doing too much.

- Develop and maintain a positive attitude. View changes as positive challenges, opportunities or blessings.

- Rehearse for stressful events. Imagine yourself feeling calm and confident in an anticipated stressful situation. You will be able to relax more easily when the situation arises.

- Modify your environment to get rid of or manage your exposure to things that cause stress.

CHAPTER 8
CHILDREN'S HEALTH

BED-WETTING

Wetting the bed is not only uncomfortable, it is also embarrassing, especially for a child older than three years. And that's not all. Fear of wetting the bed may cause children to miss out on social activities such as staying the night with friends or going camping.

Three out of four toddlers stay dry all night by age 3$^1/_2$. By age 5, one in five still wets the bed. By age 6, the numbers drop to one in 10. Just about all bed-wetting stops by the time children reach puberty. Boys are more likely than girls to wet their beds. Bed-wetting may start again during stressful times.

No one really knows what causes enuresis, the medical term for bed-wetting. From the 1930s to the 1960s, it was commonly believed that children who wet their beds had psychological problems. Today, it is suspected that bed-wetting may be caused by slow development of the nerves that control the bladder.

Bed-wetting may also be caused by a bladder that is too small to hold the urine produced during the night.

Bed-wetting is sometimes a symptom of a serious illness (e.g., diabetes or a urinary tract infection), especially if it starts in a child who has previously been dry through the night.

Questions to Ask

Does your child drink an excessive amount of fluids, pass urine more than usual during the day and night and/or show other signs such as fatigue, increased appetite and weight gain and itching around the genitals? **YES**

NO

Does your child have a fever, abdominal pain or a burning sensation when passing urine? **YES**

NO

Is your child older than 6 years and has he or she never been dry at night, or has he or she been dry at night for an extended time but is now wetting the bed again? **YES**

NO

Self-Care Procedures

Your patience and love will go a long way to help a child who wets the bed. Children have no control over this condition; they don't wet the bed on purpose. Making the child feel guilty or getting angry with him or her will only delay solving this problem. Try to be understanding and supportive.

Psychologists recommend that you simply wait for the problem to pass. Don't praise the child for a dry bed or punish him or her when it's wet. To help make life easier for your child and yourself, consider the following:

- Get your child to change the bed linen as well as his or her clothes during the night, if he or she is able to do so. Or keep a flannel-covered rubber sheet nearby so your child can put it over the wet sheets.
- Set an alarm clock two to three hours after your child falls asleep so he or she can wake up to go to the toilet.
- Make sure your child empties the bladder before getting into bed.
- Encourage your child to follow instructions, if any, that the doctor suggests, such as bladder-stretching or stream-interruption exercises, or behaviour modification devices.
- Obtain a bed-wetting alarm. (This is best suited for children 5 years and older.) Modern enuresis alarms have moisture sensors that attach directly to the underwear. At the first drop of liquid, a buzzer sounds, waking up the child. Eventually, children learn to wake up whenever they feel the urge to urinate. Newer models of these alarms can help prevent wet beds about 85 to 90 per cent of the time.

Alarms are usually available on loan from health visitors or from hospital outpatient departments.

CHICKEN POX

Chicken pox is a very contagious disease caused by a virus known as the varicella or herpes zoster virus. It is spread from child to child, and sometimes to adults, by sneezing, coughing, contaminated clothing and direct contact with open blisters. Children exposed to the virus develop chicken pox seven to 21 days later.

In most cases there are no symptoms before the rash appears. Some children, though, may be tired, have a fever and complain of stomach ache a day or two before a flat, red rash appears. The rash generally begins on the scalp, face and back, but can spread to any body surface. It is rarely seen, though, on the palms of the hands or soles of the feet. Sometimes there are also spots like small ulcers inside the mouth and in the genital area.

Within hours, the flat, red spots turn into tiny clear blisters that itch a lot. As your child scratches the blisters, serum spills out, dries and forms hard crusts that loosen and drop off about two weeks later. Since the rash appears in crops every two to six days, new red spots are often seen alongside old dried scabs. Some children have very few spots while others are covered.

Most children recover from chicken pox uneventfully in less than two weeks. Complications are rare, although chicken pox can occasionally lead to encephalitis (inflammation of the brain), meningitis or pneumonia. Children who have cancer and those who take medications such as steroids that affect the immune system are at a higher risk of complications from chicken pox. The biggest problem parents face with chicken pox, though, is infected blisters.

One attack of chicken pox usually gives your child lifelong immunity. Children rarely have a second round of chicken pox, but if it does occur, the attacks are usually very mild.

Questions to Ask

Does your child with chicken pox have a severe headache, stiff neck, convulsions, abnormal behaviour and/or continuous vomiting? **YES**

↓ NO

Is your child hard to wake, confused or having trouble breathing? **YES**

↓ NO

flowchart continued in next column

Does your child have cancer, or is your child taking drugs (e.g., steroids) that affect the immune system, and does he or she have a fever higher than 39°C (102°F)? **YES**

↓ NO

Does your child have cancer, or is your child taking drugs (e.g., steroids) that affect the immune system, but does he or she *not* have a fever higher than 39°C (102°F)? **YES**

↓ NO

Does your child have a fever higher than 39.5°C (103°F)? Or has your child had a fever higher than 39°C (102°F) for more than two days? **YES**

↓ NO

Does your child have any scabs that are red, oozing pus or bleeding? **YES**

↓ NO

Self-Care Procedures

The goals are to make your child comfortable and to reduce and relieve the itching so your child does not scratch

119

off the scabs (this could start a secondary infection and/or leave scars).

- Encourage your child not to scratch the scabs. Keep him or her busy with other activities.
- Give your child a cool bath without soap every three to four hours for the first couple of days (15 to 20 minutes at a time). Add $1/2$ cup of sodium bicarbonate to the bath water. Pat, do not rub, your child dry.
- Dip a face cloth in cool water and place it on the itchy areas.
- Apply calamine lotion for temporary relief.
- Cover an infant's hands with cotton socks if he or she is scratching the sores. Trim an older child's fingernails.
- Wash your child's hands three times a day to avoid infecting the open blisters.
- Keep your child cool and calm. Heat and sweating make the itching worse. Also, keep your child out of the sun. Additional chicken pox spots will occur on parts of the skin exposed to the sun.
- Ask your pharmacist about an over-the-counter antihistamine if the itching is severe or stops your child from sleeping.
- Give your child paracetamol suspension for the fever. *Note: Do not give aspirin, or any medication containing salicylates, to children under 12 years of age, unless directed by a doctor, due to its association with Reye's syndrome, a potentially fatal condition.*
- Give your child soft foods, cold fluids and ice lollies if he or she has sores in the mouth. Do not offer salty foods or citrus fruits that may irritate the sores.
- Reassure your child that the spots are not serious and will go away in a week or so.

COLIC

Colic in a baby is a very frustrating condition for parents to deal with. Your baby cries for hours on end for no apparent reason, tucking his or her tiny knees close to the stomach as if in severe pain. Typically, attacks start in the evening when you may be most tired and your patience thin.

Nothing seems to stop the screaming of a colicky infant – not even feeding, changing the nappy or cuddling. Take comfort, though. Colic is rarely dangerous and doesn't last a long time. It usually begins after an infant is two weeks old, peaks at about three months of age and usually ends by the fourth month.

The cause of colic is a mystery. Some paediatricians think it is due to an underdeveloped digestive tract. Others blame food allergies, wind, not enough sleep or over-sensitivity to a busy and noisy home. Still others think it is a combination of these factors. An attack of colic may end with the passage of wind or a stool.

Once in a while, colic may be an early sign of a serious medical problem. For example, in the medical condition called intussusception, the bowel becomes obstructed. A doctor can examine your baby to check for this and other medical conditions.

Prevention

- Sit your infant up at feeding time to stop him or her swallowing air.
- If breast-feeding, watch your intake of caffeine drinks like colas, coffee, cocoa and tea.
- If breast-feeding, stop eating milk products on a one-week trial basis. One study showed that when the mother stopped eating dairy foods, her baby's colic often disappeared. (If you do this, check with your doctor about taking calcium supplements.)
- Do not overheat the baby's milk.
- Make sure the bottle's teat holes are not too small. Tiny holes cause babies to swallow air as they suck on the teat.
- Make feeding time a quiet, calm time.
- Give feeds more frequently. Burp your baby more often.

Questions to Ask

Is your infant lethargic – unable to be normally active? **YES**

NO

Do you feel out of control, and are you tempted to strike or hit the baby? **YES**

NO

Is your infant vomiting, having diarrhoea or passing black or bloody stools? **YES**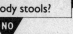

NO

flowchart continued in next column

Is your infant running a fever higher than 38.5°C (101°F)? **YES**

NO

Has your baby lost weight, or is he or she eating less or showing reluctance to feed? **YES**

NO

Is your infant younger than two weeks or older than four months? **YES**

NO

Does any attack of colic last longer than four hours? **YES**

NO

Is your infant taking a prescription drug? **YES**

NO

Self-Care Procedures

First, stay calm and try to relax. It takes a lot of patience and tolerance to deal with a screaming baby, especially when nothing seems to be wrong. While none of these Self-Care Procedures will cure colic, they may bring you and your baby some relief.

- Be sure your baby is getting enough to eat. Hunger, not colic, may be causing the crying.

- Try different types of teats. If the teat hole is too small, enlarge it.
- To check the hole size, put cold milk formula in the bottle and turn it upside down. Shake or squeeze the bottle.
- Count the number of drops of milk formula. A hole of the right size delivers about one drop per second.
- If there are fewer drops per second, make the hole bigger by using a knife to make a cross-cut over the existing hole.
- Hold your child up while feeding and for a short while afterwards.
- Burp your baby after each ounce of milk formula or every few minutes when breast-feeding.
- Use a dummy. (Never, however, put a dummy on a string around your baby's neck.)
- Wrap your infant in a cosy blanket and gently rock him or her. The back-and-forth motion tends to quiet a wailing baby.
- Try what is called the 'colic carry'. Carefully place your baby facedown, with his or her face on your open hand and his or her legs straddling your inner elbow. Support your baby by holding his or her back with your other hand and walk around the house for a while.
- Vacuum while carrying your infant in a baby sling worn on your chest. Apparently, the noise of a running vacuum soothes a colicky baby.
- Play soothing music. This may benefit you as well as the baby.
- Take your baby for a ride outdoors in his or her buggy or in the car.
- Run the dryer or dishwasher. Put your baby in an infant seat and lean it against the side of the dryer or on the worktop close to the dishwasher. (Stay with your baby and make sure the baby will not be harmed by the heat or steam given off by these appliances.) The vibration may put your child to sleep.
- Try one of the over-the-counter preparations, such as gripe water or simethicone. These sometimes help. Ask your pharmacist first.
- Let your baby cry himself or herself to sleep if none of the Self-Care Procedures works. (Don't let your baby cry, however, for more than four hours.)

CROUP

What could be more frightening than to awaken during the night to the sound of your child gasping for air and 'barking like a seal'? Yet these are the classical signs of croup, a respiratory infection that typically affects children between the ages of three months and six years. While it may sound frightening, croup is rarely cause for concern. Croup usually lasts from three to seven days. Generally, it worsens at night and tends to improve during the day.

A virus is the most common cause of croup. Infected by a virus, cells in the voice box and windpipe react by swelling up and secreting mucus that narrows these air passages. The secretions dry and thicken, making it even more difficult for your child to breathe. Dissolving the dried secretions with steam is often all that is needed to relieve your child's discomfort. Children usually outgrow croup as they get older and the windpipe becomes wider.

Sometimes croup is confused with another, more serious condition called epiglottitis (inflammation of the flap that closes the airway during swallowing). Children with epiglottitis tend to drool, tilt their heads forward, have a fever and jut their jaw out as they try to breathe. Epiglottitis has become uncommon since the introduction of Hb vaccination.

Sometimes what sounds like croup may instead indicate that your child has inhaled a foreign object. If the object blocks the windpipe, your child will have trouble breathing and will need immediate emergency care.

Questions to Ask

Is your child's breathing very laboured and is your child unable to swallow? **YES**

NO

Is your child drooling, breathing through the mouth, sticking out the chin and gasping for air? **YES**

NO

Are your child's lips and nails turning blue or dark? **YES**

NO

Self-Care Procedures

- Try not to panic. While wheezing and barking sounds are frightening, remaining calm will lessen your child's fear and anxiety.
- Hold your child to comfort him or her. Helping your child to relax may help stop the windpipe from constricting and make breathing easier.
- Use a hot bath or shower to help relieve the congestion:
  - Take your child to the bathroom and close the door.
  - Turn on the hot water in the washbasin, bath and shower to fill the room with steam.
  - Do not put your child in the shower. Instead, sit your child on the toilet or a chair, but not on the floor. Try reading a book to your child to pass the time and ease any fears.
  - Open the window to let in cool air. This helps to create more steam.
  - Allow at least 15 minutes for the steam to ease the symptoms. If this doesn't ease the breathing difficulties, see emergency care.
- Use an electric kettle to fill the child's room with steam but *never* put the kettle in reach of the child and *never* leave the child unattended.
- Crying is a good sign. It means that your child's symptoms are subsiding. A crying child is able to breathe.

FITS (CONVULSIONS OR SEIZURES)

In a fit (also known as a convulsion or seizure), abnormal electrical activity in the brain produces an altered level of consciousness and in some cases excessive shaking of the arms and legs.

Sometimes the cause of a fit is not known. There are several things, however, that are known to cause fits. Febrile convulsions are fits that occur when a child has a high fever. In fact, high fevers are the most common cause of fits in children aged six months to four years. A temperature higher than 39°C (102°F) can set off a febrile convulsion. Illnesses that cause a rapid rise in temperature, such as roseola, are often linked to febrile convulsions. A sudden high temperature seems to confuse the brain's normal electrical impulses. Fits can also occur in normal, healthy children whose internal thermometer has not fully developed.

Fits also may be triggered by poisons, infections, reactions to medications and, very rarely, by vaccinations. Even breath-holding can set off a fit. And fits are the most common symptom of epilepsy, a disorder of the brain (see p.197).

Most fits are brief, lasting from one to five minutes. Short-lasting fits do not cause permanent damage. Fits that have not stopped after 30 minutes, though, may signal a more serious condition. Any child who experiences a fit should be seen by a doctor as a matter of urgency. Less than half of the children who have a fit ever have another one.

Prevention of a febrile convulsion

The best way to prevent a febrile convulsion is rapidly to reduce the fever. This is especially important for a child who has had a febrile convulsion in the past. He or she is more likely to have another one with future fevers. Also:

- Remove most or all of your child's clothes to avoid overheating.
- Sponge your child with tepid water and give paracetamol as soon as you notice the fever. Continue trying to reduce the fever in this way until it is 38.5°C (101°F) or less. *Note: Do not give aspirin, or any medication containing salicylates, to children under 12 years of age, unless directed by a doctor, due to its association with Reye's syndrome, a potentially fatal condition.*

Questions to Ask

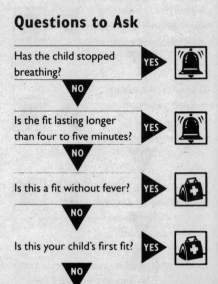

Has the child stopped breathing? **YES**

NO

Is the fit lasting longer than four to five minutes? **YES**

NO

Is this a fit without fever? **YES**

NO

Is this your child's first fit? **YES**

NO

flowchart continued on next page

Is your child younger than six months or older than four years? YES

NO

Self-Care Procedures

It is easy to panic when watching a child have a fit. Try to remember, though, that if it is a febrile convulsion, it will stop by itself within a few minutes. The primary concern should be preventing injury to the child during the fit and lowering his or her temperature.

- During the fit, protect the child from falling and hitting his or her head on a table edge or any sharp object. Move furniture, toys and other objects out of the way.
- Make sure his or her air passage is open.
  - Gently pull on the jaw as you extend the neck backwards.
  - Roll the child on his or side to allow saliva to drain from the mouth.
  - Clear the mouth of vomit, if there is any, so the child can breathe.
- Do not force anything into a child's mouth to prevent him or her from biting the tongue. Children rarely bite their tongues during a febrile convulsion.
- Give your child rectal diazepam if your doctor has prescribed this to stop a febrile convulsion.
- If the fit is due to a fever, start lowering your child's temperature as soon as the fit subsides by sponging the body with

water at room temperature. Do not put the child in the bath. Do not use an ice pack because it lowers the temperature too quickly.
- Do not give medication, foods or fluids by mouth during a fit.
- Note how many minutes the fit lasts and observe the symptoms that take place so you can report these to the doctor.
- Following the fit, the child will probably be sleepy and not remember what has happened. This is normal.
- Leave the child without clothes if possible, put him or her in a cool room to sleep and call your doctor.

LICE

Head lice are tiny parasites 2–3 mm (about $^1/_{10}$ in long). These flat, wingless creatures survive by sucking human blood. Louse bites cause an intense itching and red spots on the skin that look like mosquito bites. The adult lice are rarely seen. Instead, you see what are called nits, clusters of lice eggs, which are white and about the size of a pin head. They are deposited on hair strands and often mistaken for dandruff.

Lice spread quickly from person to person. No matter how well-groomed and clean your child is, he or she can get them from anyone who already has them. Female lice lay eggs every day. The eggs hatch in eight to 10 days, after which they soon begin their annoying biting.

There are three types of lice: head lice, body lice and pubic lice. All are very attracted to body heat. Head lice are the most common type, especially among children. Body lice live in the seams of dirty clothes and bedding. Pubic lice, which are found on the pubic hair, are sexually transmitted and commonly called 'crabs' because the lice look like crabs.

Prevention

To prevent head lice, children should be told:
- Do not share hats, brushes or combs.
- Do not lie on a pillow shared with another child.
- Comb hair frequently.
You should:
- Change bed linen often and wash it in hot water, especially during an epidemic of lice at school.
- Vacuum furniture, mattresses, rugs, stuffed animals and car seats if anyone in your family is infected with lice. Do not use insecticidal sprays for lice.
- Immediately notify anyone who may have been in close contact with your child to help prevent infecting others with lice. Be sure to tell:
  - Your child's school
  - Your child-minder or nanny
  - Parents of your child's friends
- Wash combs and brushes. Then soak them in hot, not boiling, water for 10 minutes.
- Check your children for head lice and nits at least once a week. Check more often if your child is scratching his or her head. Look for nits around the nape of the neck and behind the ears.

Questions to Ask

Are there open wounds on your child's scalp caused by scratching? **YES**

NO

Have you found lice or nits in your child's eyebrows or eyelashes or on the hair shaft or skin? **YES**

NO

Does your child's scalp itch, do you see red bite marks, and are lymph glands in the neck swollen? **YES**

NO

If your child has lice, does he or she have allergies or other health problems, or is your child under two years of age? **YES**

NO

Self-Care Procedures

Only insecticidal lotions and shampoos kill lice. You can buy these products at a chemists without a prescription. Lotions are generally more effective than shampoos but you may not be able to use them on family members with eczema (check with your doctor or health visitor). All lice-killing products are pesticides:

consequently, they must be used with caution and only as directed.

Everyone in your household should be checked for lice and nits. Treat all the family at the same time even if some family members appear not to be infested.

When using an insecticidal product:
- Follow the directions exactly as given.
- Avoid using a hair dryer as this reduces the effectiveness.

Other tips:
- There is no need to remove nits, but if you want to do so for cosmetic reasons, this is most easily done with a nit comb obtainable from chemists.
- Soak all combs and brushes in insecticidal lotion or for 10 minutes in hot water.
- Immediately wash bedding and clothing in water hotter than 50°C (125°F). Heat kills the lice and destroys the nits.
- Dry-clean clothing and hats that cannot be washed.

MEASLES

Measles is a very contagious disease caused by the rubeola virus. It mostly occurs in children, but can affect older persons, too. With proper immunization, though, the disease is preventable. Current recommendations in the UK are for children to be given a single measles, mumps, rubella (MMR) immunization when they are 13 months old. Given this immunization, your child will probably never get measles. So make sure he or she is immunized.

When a child does get measles, he or she has probably been exposed to someone else who had it 10 to 12 days earlier. The symptoms of measles usually develp in this order:
- Temperature of 39°C (102°F) or higher
- Fatigue
- Loss of appetite
- Runny nose and sneezing
- Cough
- Red eyes and sensitivity to light
- Tiny white spots (called Koplik spots) in the mouth and throat
- Blotchy red rash that starts on the face and spreads to the rest of the body: to the chest and abdomen and then to the arms and legs. The rash usually lasts for up to seven days.

The measles virus is spread by nose, mouth or throat secretions, either on soiled articles or through coughing, sneezing and so on. It can be passed on three to six days before the rash appears as well as up to seven days after the rash starts.

If your child has been exposed to measles, but hasn't been immunized, contact your GP. If given early enough, a measles vaccine may prevent your child from getting measles. An injection of gamma globulin can help protect against measles for three months. Let your child's school know if your child has measles.

If your child gets measles, not much can be done to shorten the illness. He or she will probably start feeling better by the fourth day of the rash unless other problems occur. Possible complications include eye or ear infections, pneumonia and meningitis.

Questions to Ask

Are any of these problems present:
- Blue or purple lips or nails
- Convulsions
- Extreme difficulty in breathing
- Unable to speak more than three or four words between breaths
- Confusion or excessive drowsiness
- Severe headache and stiff neck
- Bleeding from the nose or mouth or into the skin
- Dark purple blotches on the skin

YES

NO

Are any of these problems present:
- Sore throat
- Earache or tugging at the ears
- A yellow discharge from the eyes or nose
- Breathing that is laboured, but not due to a stuffy nose
- Fever that comes back after temperature has been normal for a day or more or fever that is still present beyond the fourth day of the rash

YES

NO

Self-Care Procedures

- Keep a record of your child's temperature. Take it in the morning and the evening. Give the recommended dose of paracetamol for fever and/or aches and pains. *Note: Do not give aspirin, or any medication containing salicylates, to children under 12 years of age, unless directed by a doctor, due to its association with Reye's syndrome, a potentially fatal condition.*
- Isolate your child from other people who have not had measles or a measles immunization. Any child who has come in contact with your child should be taken for a measles immunization unless he or she has already been immunized or had measles.
- Because your child's eyes may be sensitive:
  - Keep the lighting in the house dim. Draw the curtains, pull the blinds down and use low-wattage light bulbs.
  - If your child must go outdoors, get him or her to wear sunglasses.
  - Keep the TV and video games turned off.
  - Urge your child not to read or do close-up work.
  - Wipe your child's closed eyes with a clean wet cloth or ball of cotton wool several times a day.
  For a cough:
  - Give steam inhalations, especially at night.
  - If your child is five years of age or older, give him or her cough drops, lozenges or boiled sweets to suck.
  - Give your child plenty of fluids. Water is helpful in loosening mucus and also

soothes an irritated throat. Fruit juices, fizzy drinks and tea are also good.

- Give your child cough medicines as recommended by his or her doctor or pharmacist.
- You can make your own cough medicine at home by mixing one part lemon juice and two parts honey. (Do not give to children under one year of age.)
- Get your child to rest until the fever and rash go away.
- Keep your child home from school for at least seven days after the start of the rash. It will probably be longer than this before he or she is fully recovered.

SKIN RASHES

Skin rashes come in all forms and sizes. Some are raised bumps; others are flat red blotches. Some are itchy blisters; others are patches of rough skin. Most rashes are harmless and clear up on their own within a few days, but a few may need medical attention.

The chart on p. 51 lists information on some common skin rashes.

Questions to Ask

Does your child have a reddish purple, blotchy rash which doesn't fade when you press on it? **YES**

NO

flowchart continued in next column

Does the child have any of the following:
- Fever
- Headache
- Sore throat
- A fine red rash that feels rough like sandpaper
- Joint pain along with a rash that looks like lots of small targets

YES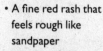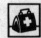

NO

Are there any large, fluid-filled blisters present or pus or swelling around the spots?

YES

NO

Has your child recently been exposed to someone with a severe sore throat?

YES

NO

If your child has nappy rash, are there also blisters or small red patches outside the nappy area, such as on the chest?

YES

NO

When the rash started, was the child taking any medications or was he or she stung by an insect?

YES

NO

flowchart continued on next page

Is your child's rash getting worse, keeping him or her from sleeping and/or do Self-Care Procedures not relieve symptoms? **YES**

NO

Self-Care Procedures

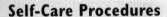

Nappy rash is best treated as follows:
• Change nappies as soon as they become wet or soiled (even at night).
• Wash your baby with plenty of warm water, not disposable wipes, to prevent irritating the skin. If the skin appears irritated, apply a light coat of zinc oxide ointment after the skin is completely dry.
• Keep the skin dry and exposed to air.
• Keep your baby's bottom uncovered, on a soft, fluffy towel, for 10 to 15 minutes before putting on a clean nappy.
• Put nappies on loosely so air can circulate under them. Avoid disposable nappies with tight leg bands.
• Don't use plastic pants until the rash is gone.
• Wash cloth nappies in mild soap. Add $1/2$ cup of vinegar to your rinse water to help remove what's left of the soap.
   Cradle cap can be treated with an anti-dandruff shampoo. Use it once a day, massaging your baby's scalp with a soft brush or face cloth for five minutes. You can soften the hard crusts of this rash by applying olive oil to the scalp overnight

before washing your child's hair. Be sure to wash the oil out thoroughly; otherwise, the cradle cap may worsen.

   Heat rash is best treated by keeping your child in a cool, dry area. It will usually disappear within two to three days if you keep the skin cool. You can ease your child's discomfort if you:
• Give him or her a bath in cool water, without soap, every couple of hours.
• Let your child's skin air dry.
• Apply calamine lotion to the very itchy spots.
• Avoid ointments and creams that can block the sweat gland pores.
   Hives (nettle rash) can be eased if you:
• Give your child an antihistamine such as Benadryl. Remember, though, that most antihistamines are likely to make your child drowsy.
• Cool your child down. Hold a wrapped ice pack over the hives, drape a face cloth dipped in cool water over the affected areas or give a cool-water bath.
• Apply calamine lotion, witch hazel or zinc oxide to the rash.
• Find and eliminate the cause of the allergic reaction.

SWOLLEN GLANDS

The lymphatic system, an important part of the immune system, is made up of numerous lymph glands (also called nodes) and the lymph channels that connect them. When a virus or other organism invades the body, the lymph glands set to work, sending out one type of white blood cell ready to kill the invaders. Lymph glands also act as filters, trapping viruses, bacteria and cancer cells.

Normally, you cannot feel your child's lymph glands except when they swell in response to an infection or foreign body. As a general rule, infections cause swollen lymph glands that are tender to the touch. The nodes often stay enlarged long after the infection is gone. In fact, most visits to the doctor for swollen glands occur after parents notice a neck node that has been present for a while. These nodes are generally painless and harmless. Be aware, though, that when the nodes are hard and rubbery and are increasing in size, they may, very rarely, be caused by a more serious disease such as lymphoma (cancer of the lymph glands), leukaemia or other type of cancer.

The salivary glands are not lymph glands. The salivary glands are not part of the immune system, but may become swollen in response to infection with the mumps virus. The salivary glands are found under the tongue, on the floor of the mouth and just below the ear lobe. It is the salivary glands located under the ear lobe, close to the jaw line, that swell when invaded by the mumps virus.

Causes of Swollen Lymph Glands

• Infections in the throat and/or ear are the most common causes of swollen glands in the neck. Infections in the feet, legs and genital area cause lymph glands to swell in the groin.

• Infectious mononucleosis, also known as glandular fever
• Rubella (German measles)
• Insect bites
• Recent dental treatment
• Lymphoma (a cancer of the lymph glands) or leukaemia
• Tuberculosis (TB)

Prevention

• Make sure your children's immunizations against measles, mumps and rubella (MMR) are up-to-date.
• Keep your child away from people you know to have contagious conditions.

Questions to Ask

Are the swollen glands tender and located at the bottom of the neck? YES

NO

Has your child had swollen glands for more than three weeks without apparent cause? YES

NO

Does your child also have a sore throat and/or fever? YES

NO

flowchart continued on next page

Are the swollen glands obvious between the jaw and under the ear? (This could be mumps.) **YES**

NO

Are the enlarged glands towards the back of the neck, and is there a pink rash on the face? (This could be rubella.) **YES**

NO

Are the swollen glands 2–3 cm (1 in) or more in diameter? **YES**

NO

Self-Care Procedures

There is little you can do for swollen glands except to treat the underlying cause. Watch to see if the glands enlarge or if others swell as well. If the swollen glands continue to enlarge or last more than three or four weeks, it's a good idea to consult your doctor.

You can, however, make your child more comfortable if you:

- Encourage him or her to rest when tired and to avoid activities that may cause more fatigue.
- Give your child lots of liquids to drink.
- Wash any scratches or other injuries thoroughly. Also apply antiseptic cream and a warm compress if necessary.

See also: 'Self-Care Procedures for Measles' on page 127, for 'Sore Throats' on page 17 and for 'Tonsillitis' on page 132.

TONSILLITIS

The tonsils are masses of tissue at each side of the back of the throat. They act as a filter to help prevent infections in the throat, mouth and sinuses from spreading to other parts of the body. They also produce antibodies that fight throat and nose infections. Tonsillitis is the medical name for inflammation of the tonsils, which may be caused by a bacterial or viral infection.

Symptoms of tonsillitis include:

- Mild to severe throat pain
- Swollen lymph glands on either side of the neck or jaw
- Ear pain
- Difficulty in swallowing
- Chills and fever
- Headache

It can be very difficult to say whether a sore throat is caused by a bacterial or a viral infection. In some cases your GP might want to take a throat swab to find out for sure. Antibiotics will only help with bacterial infections.

More often than not, having tonsillitis, does not mean that the tonsils need to be removed (in a surgical procedure called a tonsillectomy). This used to be a very common operation but these days it is recommended for only a few children. If your child has had tonsillitis more than four times in a year or has had an abscess on the tonsils your GP will probably refer your child to an ears, nose and throat (ENT) surgeon for his opinion.

Questions to Ask

Is the tonsillitis severe and/or are these problems present?
- Extreme difficulty in swallowing
- Inability to swallow saliva
- Difficulty in breathing
- Inability to say more than three to four words between breaths
- Drooling

YES

NO

Is your child unable to open fully his or her mouth?

YES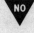

NO

Does your child have large tonsils that:
- Touch each other when not infected, or
- Result in continued mouth breathing, or
- Cause his or her speech to be muffled

YES

NO

flowchart continued in next column

Do any of the following accompany your child's tonsillitis:
- Fever
- Swollen, enlarged or tender neck glands
- Headache
- Ear pain or tugging at the ears
- Bad breath
- Loss of appetite
- Vomiting or abdominal pain

YES

NO

Do the tonsils or back of the throat look bright red or have visible pus deposits?

YES

NO

Does someone else in the family have a severe sore throat or does your child get tonsillitis often?

YES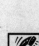

NO

Has your child's sore throat lasted more than two weeks even though it is mild?

YES

NO

Self-Care Procedures

You can take steps to relieve discomfort from tonsillitis. Get your child to:

- Gargle every few hours with a solution of $1/4$ teaspoon of salt dissolved in about 15 centilitres ($1/4$ pint) of warm water. (Children under about eight years old will not be able to manage this.)
- Drink plenty of warm drinks such as tea and soup, if tolerated.
- Eat foods that are soft and/or cold and easy to swallow (e.g., juices, ice cream and lollies). Avoid spicy foods.
- Suck on a boiled sweet or medicated lozenge occasionally (if your child is five years of age or older).
- Take the recommended dosage of paracetamol for pain and/or fever. *Note: Do not give aspirin, or any medication containing salicylates, to children under 12 years of age, unless directed by a doctor, due to its association with Reye's syndrome, a potentially fatal condition.*
- Avoid throat sprays. These may contain benzocaine, which could cause an adverse reaction.
- Avoid cigarette smoke.

WHEEZING

Wheezing is a high-pitched purring or whistling sound. It is heard more on breathing out than on breathing in. The wheezing sound is usually caused by air flowing through swollen and narrowed breathing tubes that are in spasm. Muscle spasms in the airways make breathing even more difficult.

Wheezing is sometimes confused with other respiratory sounds. The sounds of croup, for example, resemble a harsh, raspy noise on breathing in and are sometimes accompanied by a high-pitched cough. A stuffed nose, though, emits a snorting sound. And a rattling sound is often due to mucus in the windpipe.

Consider wheezing as a warning sign that your child is having trouble breathing. It is a good idea to check with your doctor if your child wheezes.

Causes of Wheezing

- Asthma, which is often a disease of childhood. More than half of the affected youngsters outgrow asthma by the time they become adults, though it can recur later in life. Asthma attacks can be frightening for parent and child alike. Many things can trigger an asthma attack such as:
  - Exposure to something your child is allergic to, including dust mites, pollen, mould, food, animal dander (flakes of dead skin) and perfume.
  - Exercise.
  - Medications.
  - Stressful event.
  - Change in the weather, especially a rapid rise or fall in barometric pressure and temperature.
  - Noxious fumes from wet paint, disinfectants, pesticides, tobacco smoke, burning coals, vehicle exhaust, wood smoke and similar smells, to name a few.
  - Ice cold drinks or cold air. Breathing tubes sometimes constrict when exposed to extreme cold.
  - Respiratory infection (bacterial or viral, especially in infants).

- Other possible causes of wheezing include:
  - Foreign objects caught in the airway.
  - Severe allergic reaction.
  - Pneumonia, acute bronchitis or congestive heart failure.
  - Genetic disorders that affect the lungs.

Questions to Ask

(Note: You may need to do the Heimlich manoeuvre (for choking) or cardiopulmonary resuscitation (CPR), and also call 999, if your child is turning blue and/or not breathing. Attend emergency first aid classes to learn when and how to do each of these procedures.)

Is your child turning blue and/or not breathing? **YES**

NO

Perform CPR if trained and Seek Emergency Care.

Did your child's wheezing start during the past few hours and is he or she coughing up bubbly, pink or white phlegm? **YES**

NO

flowchart continued in next column

Does your child look like he or she is suffocating or have severe wheezing or shortness of breath and is he or she unable to speak or drink? **YES**

NO

Does your child have a fever above 38.5°C (101°F)? **YES**

NO

If your child has asthma, is the wheezing getting worse and/or not responding to treatment? **YES**

NO

Self-Care procedures

While there is no cure for viral infections, allergic reactions and asthma, you can ease your child's wheezing in many ways:
- Encourage your child to drink plenty of fluids to thin the mucus. Coax your child to sip juice, water, or weak tea. Do not give your child ice cold drinks.
- Carry your child to the bathroom and turn on the hot water taps in the washbasin, bath and shower. (See 'Self-Care Procedures for Croup' on page 123.)

For a child suffering from an asthma attack:

135

- Remain calm.
- Follow the home treatment recommended by your doctor.
- Get your child to use his or her bronchodilator, as instructed by the doctor.
- If the asthma attack is caused by an allergic reaction, find ways to reduce your child's exposure to the allergens that triggered the attack.

If your child has asthma, the following tips might reduce the frequency of attacks:
- Prepare a solution of bleach ($^3/_4$ cup of bleach per gallon of water) and wipe bathroom tiles and floors, kitchen appliances, woodwork and anywhere else fungus and mould may be growing. Then air out the room.
- Pet dander (flakes of dead skin) sets off allergic reactions in many children. If your child is allergic to cats or dogs, try to keep the animals outside or away from your child, but especially out of the bedroom.
- Vacuum often to suck up dust mites, pollen and pet dander. Avoid disturbing dust when your child is around.
- Cover your child's mattress and pillow in plastic to avoid exposure to dust mites that like to hide in the creases.
- If you smoke, stop. Even residual smoke in a room can trigger an attack.
- Use washable rugs instead of carpeting. Carpeting is like a magnet to pollen, pet dander, mould and dust mites; its fibres attract these allergens.
- Use pillows and duvets with polyester fibres, not feathers, and wash them often.

If the asthma attack is caused by exercise, get your child to:
- Avoid exercising in cold weather.
- Swim, because pool areas are usually humid.
- Start out slowly and pace him- or herself during the activity to avoid an attack.
- Take prescribed medication about 15 minutes before exercising.
- Shower, wash his or her hair and put on clean clothes after coming in contact with grass, pollen, animals or other substances he or she is allergic to.

(Note: Keep small objects, such as detachable toy parts and foods, such as peanuts and popcorn, out of the reach of small children, to prevent them from inhaling them.)

CHAPTER 9
WOMEN'S HEALTH

BREAST CANCER AND BREAST SELF-EXAMINATION

Breast cancer is the most common form of cancer among women. One woman in 12 will develop the disease at some time in her life. Each year, about 14,000 women in England and Wales die from the disease. Most of these women are over 65 years old. Men can also develop breast cancer, but it is very unusual.

Breast cancer is a malignant tumour which invades and destroys normal tissue. When the tumor breaks away and spreads to other parts of the body, it is called a metastasis. Breast cancers can spread to the lymph nodes, lungs, liver, bone and brain.

The risk of breast cancer increases above the normal risk with these factors:
- Having had cancer in one breast, which increases the risk for cancer in the other breast
- Never giving birth or giving birth after age 30
- Early onset of menstruation (before age 12)
- Late menopause (after age 55)
- Family history of breast cancer, especially for mothers, daughters and sisters of women with breast cancer prior to the menopause
- Exposure to radiation
- Diet high in fat
- Obesity
- Diabetes
- Recent injury

Detection

Any woman who notices a lump in her breast or any of the other symptoms mentioned previously should see her doctor as soon as possible.

In the UK, mammograms to screen for breast cancer are offered on the NHS at three-yearly intervals to women between the ages of 50 to 65. Mammograms are also offered on the NHS to younger women with a family history of breast cancer. The interpretation of mammograms in younger women is more difficult as breast tissue is denser. Ultrasound can be useful in these cases, particularly for diagnosing cysts.

Cells from a suspicious lump can be withdrawn through a very fine biopsy needle and tested to see if they are malignant.

Treatment

There are a variety of treatments for breast cancer. The main treatment is surgery. The removal of the cancerous area is most often recommended along with taking a sample of the lymph nodes in the armpit to see if cancer has spread there. Other treatments are radiotherapy, chemotherapy and hormonal therapy.

It is important to find out the type of cancer cell that is involved. If the cancer is a type that spreads quickly, a more extensive surgical treatment may be chosen.

Types of Surgical Procedures:

Lumpectomy – The lump and an area of surrounding tissue are removed.

Partial or segmental mastectomy – The tumour and up to one-quarter of the breast tissue are removed.

Simple or total mastectomy – The entire breast is removed.

Modified radical mastectomy – The entire breast, the underarm lymph nodes and the lining covering the chest muscles, but not the muscles themselves, are removed.

Radical mastectomy – The breast, lymph nodes in the armpit and the chest muscles under the breast are removed. (This operation is now performed only very rarely.)

Ask your doctor about the benefits and risks for each surgical option and decide together which option is best for you.

Questions to Ask

Can you see or feel any lumps, thickening or changes of any kind when you examine your breasts? For example, is there dimpling, puckering or retraction of the skin or a change in the shape or contour of the breast?

YES

NO

Do you have breast pain or a constant tenderness that lasts throughout the menstrual cycle?

YES

NO

If you normally have lumpy breasts (already diagnosed as being non-cancerous by your doctor), can you see or feel any new lumps or have any lumps changed in size? Or are you concerned about having non-cancerous lumps?

YES

NO

Do the nipples become drawn into the chest or totally inverted, change shape or become crusty from a discharge?

YES

NO

flowchart continued on next page

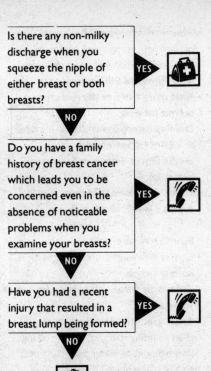

Is there any non-milky discharge when you squeeze the nipple of either breast or both breasts?

YES

NO

Do you have a family history of breast cancer which leads you to be concerned even in the absence of noticeable problems when you examine your breasts?

YES

NO

Have you had a recent injury that resulted in a breast lump being formed?

YES

NO

Self-Care Procedures

How to Examine Your Breasts

It is normal to have some lumpiness or thickening in the breasts. By examining your breasts regularly, you will learn what is normal for you and when any changes do occur. The more you examine your breasts, the better you can learn what is normal for you. Your 'job' isn't just to find lumps, but also to notice if there are any changes.

In the shower – With your fingers flat, move gently over every part of each breast. Use your right hand to examine the left breast and your left hand to examine the right breast. Check for any thickening, hard lump or knot.

In front of a mirror – Check your breasts with your arms at your sides. Then raise your arms overhead. Look for any changes in the shape of each breast, swelling, dimpling or changes in the nipples.

Lying down – To examine your right breast, put a pillow under your right shoulder. Place your right hand behind your head. Keeping the fingers of your left hand flat, press gently in small circular motions around an imaginary clock face. Begin at the outermost top of your right breast for 12 o'clock, then move to 10 o'clock, and so on, until you get back to 12 o'clock. Each breast will have a normal ridge of firm tissue. Then move in 2–3 cm (1 in) towards the nipple. Keep circling to examine every part of your breast, including the nipple.

Repeat the procedure on the left breast with a pillow under the left shoulder and your left hand behind your head. Finally, squeeze the nipple of each breast gently between the thumb and index finger. Any discharge, clear or bloody, should be reported to your doctor immediately.

EATING DISORDERS: ANOREXIA NERVOSA AND BULIMIA

An eating disorder may be defined, in a sense, as self-abuse. It can be just as harmful to your health as substance abuse involving alcohol or drugs. Two of these disorders, anorexia and bulimia, result from the fear of overeating and of gaining weight. They also share other common traits that reflect the mental and physical health of the sufferer:

• Depression
• Low self-esteem, poor body image
• Self-destructive outlook, self-punishment for some imagined wrong
• Disturbed family relationships
• Increased rate of illness due to low weight, frequent weight gain/loss and/or poor nutrition
• Abnormal preoccupation with food and with feeling out of control

In addition, anorexia and bulimia have factors specific to each:
Anorexia nervosa sufferers:
• Are usually pre-teenage or teenage females.
• Grow up in 'over-achieving' families who establish unusually high expectations for their children.
• Place exaggerated emphasis on body image and perfection.
• Have parents who are very busy and involved in their own lives. The anorexic may feel the need to be perfect to gain parental attention.

• Have marked physical effects: loss of head hair, stoppage of ovulation/menstruation, slowed heart rate, low blood pressure and intolerance to cold.
• Have more extreme depression than bulimia patients.
• Develop osteoporosis later in life due to lack of calcium and decreased production of oestrogen if menstruation stops.
• Have severe damage to heart and vital organs if weight drops sufficiently.

Bulimia sufferers:
• Can be overweight, underweight or normal weight.
• Are mostly female, older teenagers or young adults.
• Are characterized by binge eating and then vomiting (purging) and/or taking laxatives and/or water pills (diuretics) to 'undo' the binge.
• Have severe health problems that arise from a binge-purge cycle of eating. These include tears in the stomach lining, irregular heartbeat, kidney damage from low potassium levels, damage to tooth enamel from vomited stomach acids and cessation of menstruation.
• Repress anger from inability to express emotions in an assertive way. They fear upsetting important people in their lives.

There is no one cause for these eating disorders. Many factors contribute to them:
• A possible genetic predisposition.
• Social pressure to be thin.
• Personal or family pressures.

- Metabolic and biochemical problems or abnormalities.

Treatment for anorexia and/or bulimia includes:
- Medical diagnosis and care, the earlier the better.
- Psychotherapy, individual, family and/or group.
- Behaviour therapy.
- Medication. Antidepressant medicine is sometimes used.
- Nutrition therapy, including vitamin and mineral supplements.
- Hospitalization, if necessary, especially in anorexia, if weight has dropped about 25 per cent or more below normal weight and/or has affected vital functions.

Questions to Ask

Have you reached a weight that is 15 per cent less than what is standard for your age and height by intentionally dieting and exercising (not due to any known illness)? **YES**

NO

flowchart continued in next column

Do you have any of these problems:
- Irregular heartbeat
- Slow pulse, low blood pressure
- Low body temperature, cold hands and feet
- Thin hair (or hair loss) on the head, baby-like hair on the body (lanugo)
- Dry skin, fingernails that split, peel or crack
- Problems with digestion, bloating, constipation
- Three or more missed periods (in a row), delayed onset of menstruation, infertility
- Sometimes depression and lethargy, sometimes euphoria and hyperactivity
- Tiredness, weakness, muscle cramps, tremors
- Lack of concentration

YES

NO

Do you have an intense fear of gaining weight or of getting fat or see yourself as fat even though you are of normal weight or are underweight? Do you continue to diet and exercise excessively even though you have reached your goal weight? **YES**

NO

flowchart continued on next page

Are you aware that your eating pattern is not normal and are you afraid that you will not be able to stop binge eating? Are you depressed after bingeing on food?

YES

NO

Do you:
- Hoard food
- Leave the table straight after meals to go to the toilet to induce vomiting and/or spend long periods of time in the toilet as a result of taking laxatives and/or water pills (diuretics)

YES

NO

flowchart continued in next column

Do you have recurrent episodes when you eat a large amount of food in less than two hours time at a very fast pace, and do you do at least three of the following:
- Eat high calorie, easily consumed food during a binge
- Binge eat with no one watching
- Stop the binge eating when you get abdominal pain, go to sleep, interact socially or induce vomiting
- Attempt to lose weight repeatedly with very strict diets, self-induced vomiting and/or laxatives or water pills (diuretics)
- Have weight changes of more than 4.5 kg (10 lb) due to bingeing and fasting

YES

NO

Self-Care Procedures

Eating disorders are too complicated and physically hazardous to be treated with self-care procedures. Experts agree that experienced professionals should treat people who have eating disorders.

But to avoid succumbing to an eating disorder, follow these suggestions:

- Accept yourself and your body. You don't need to be or look like anyone else. Spend time with people who accept you as you are, not people who focus exclusively on thinness.
- Eat a wholesome nutritious diet. Focus on complex carbohydrates (e.g., whole grains and beans), fresh fruits and vegetables, low-fat dairy foods and low-fat meats.
- Eat at regular times during the day. Don't skip meals. If you do so, you are more likely to binge when you do eat.
- Avoid refined foods (e.g., white flour and sugar) and 'junk' foods high in calories, fat and sugar (e.g., cakes, biscuits or pastries). Bulimics tend to binge on junk food. The more they eat, the more they want.
- Get regular moderate exercise. If you find that you are exercising excessively, make an effort to get involved in non-exercise activities with friends and family.
- Find success in things that you do. Your work, hobbies and volunteer activities will promote self-esteem.
- Educate yourself. Learn as much as you can about eating disorders from books and organizations that deal with them.
- Parents who want to help daughters avoid eating disorders should promote a balance between their daughters' competing needs for both independence and family involvement.

ENDOMETRIOSIS

Endometriosis is an abnormal condition that occurs when growth of the tissue that lines the inside of the uterus (endometrium) is found outside of the uterus in other areas of the body. This misplaced tissue undergoes the same cyclical changes that occur in the lining of the uterus during menstruation. Endometriosis can only occur after menstruation begins in a woman. Women in their 20s, 30s and 40s are most likely to get endometriosis.

The most common symptoms of endometriosis are:
- Abdominal pain before and during menstrual periods (usually worse than the pain in normal menstrual cramps)
- Pain during or after sexual intercourse
- Painful urination
- Lower back pain and/or painful bowel movements during menstrual periods
- Pelvic soreness/tenderness
  Pain, however, is not always present.
Other symptoms include:
- Abnormally heavy or long menstrual periods
- Infertility

The exact cause of endometriosis is unknown. One theory suggests that some of the fluid and tissue shed during menstruation goes back up the fallopian tubes and out into the peritoneal cavity rather than being lost through the vagina. This tissue then seeds itself around the pelvis. Other theories point to problems with the immune system and/or hormones. There is also some evidence that the condition may be inherited.

Places where endometriosis is commonly found are:
- Outside surface of the uterus
- Fallopian tubes
- Ovaries
- Lining of the pelvic cavity
- Area between the vagina and the rectum

A GP will often suspect that a woman has endometriosis. This provisional diagnosis will be confirmed by a gynaecologist. The gynaecologist may perform a laparoscopy, which is an outpatient surgical procedure, performed under general anaesthetic, in which a slim telescope is inserted through a very small opening made in the navel. This allows the doctor to examine the pelvic organs and evaluate the extent of the disease.

The management of endometriosis is aimed at suppressing levels of the hormones oestrogen and progesterone. These hormones cause endometriosis to grow. Mild to moderate endometriosis may cause few symptoms after the menopause but may be reactivated by HRT.

Treatment for endometriosis can include surgery or drugs. Surgical treatment can be a conservative approach, such as removing areas of endometriosis through a laparoscope using laser, cautery or small surgical instruments to destroy the growths. These treatments are used to reduce pain and to increase fertility in some women.

More radically, surgery may be performed to remove some or all of the affected pelvic organs. This will usually relieve symptoms and may be an appropriate option for a woman who does not wish to have children.

Drug treatment consists of:
- Painkillers, as well as antiprostaglandins (e.g., ibuprofen).
- Oral contraceptives, which temporarily stop ovulation and menstruation. These are more likely to be used for very mild cases of endometriosis.
- Anti-oestrogens, such as danazol, which suppress a woman's production of oestrogen. This treatment will stop the menstrual cycle and prevent further growth of endometriosis since endometriosis needs oestrogen to grow. These drugs can have side effects such as acne, hair growth on the face and changes in the libido.
- Progesterone, which suppresses the growth of endometrial cells.
- Gonadotropin-releasing hormone (GnRH) agonist drugs, which will inhibit the production of oestrogen. This therapy causes a medically induced menopause that is temporary.

Questions to Ask

Do you have a lot of pain:
- During sex
- When you menstruate and has this worsened over time
- When you urinate

YES

 NO

flowchart continued on next page

Have you tried to get pregnant, but have not succeeded after 12 or more months? **YES**

NO

Self-Care Procedures

Self-Care Procedures are very limited for endometriosis. It needs medical treatment. Things you can do to enhance medical treatment include:

• Exercise regularly.

• Eat a diet high in nutrients and low in fat, especially saturated fat, mostly found in coconut and palm oils, animal sources of fat and hydrogenated vegetable fats.

• Take aspirin, paracetamol or ibuprofen for pain. Check with your doctor for his or her preference. *Note: Do not give aspirin, or any medication containing salicylates, to children under 12 years of age, unless directed by a doctor, due to its association with Reye's syndrome, a potentially fatal condition.*

• Consider using oral contraceptives for birth control. Women who take the pill have a reduced incidence of endometriosis.

FIBROIDS

Fibroids are benign (non-cancerous) tumours formed mostly of muscle tissue. They are found in the wall of the uterus and sometimes on the cervix. They can range in size from as small as a pea to as large as a football. With larger fibroids, a woman's uterus can grow to the size it reaches after 20 weeks of pregnancy. About 20 to 25 per cent of women over 35 get fibroids. A woman is more likely to get fibroids if:

• She has not been pregnant.

• She has a close relative who also has or has had them.

• She is of Afro-Caribbean origin. The risk is three to five times higher than it is for Caucasian women.

Why fibroids occur is not really known. They do, however, depend on oestrogen for their growth. They may shrink or even disappear after the menopause.

Symptoms of Fibroids

Some women with uterine fibroids do not have any symptoms or problems from them. When symptoms or problems do occur, they vary due to the number, size and locations of the fibroid(s). Possible symptoms and problems include:

• Heavy menstrual bleeding

• Abdominal swelling especially if the fibroids are large

• Pain (backache, during sex, during periods), from pressure on the internal organs

145

- Anaemia from excessive bleeding
- Frequent urination due to pressure on the bladder
- Chronic constipation due to pressure on the rectum
- Infertility, because the fallopian tubes may be blocked or the uterus may be distorted
- Miscarriage, because if the fibroid is inside the uterus, the placenta may not implant as it should

You can find out if you have fibroids when your doctor takes a medical history and performs a pelvic examination. A doctor can also do other tests to confirm their presence, location and size. An ultrasound is the most common test for diagnosing fibroids.

Treatments for fibroids include:

- 'Watchful waiting' if they are small, harmless and painless or not causing any problems. Your doctor will 'watch' for any changes and may suggest 'waiting' for the menopause, since fibroids often shrink or disappear after that time. If you have problems during this 'waiting' period (e.g., too much pain, too much bleeding, your abdomen gets too big, you have to take daily iron supplements to prevent anaemia or you have gastrointestinal problems), you may decide that you do not want to 'wait' for the menopause, but instead choose to have something done to treat your fibroids.
- Medication. One type called gonadotropin-releasing hormone (GnRH) agonists blocks the production of oestrogen by the ovaries. This

shrinks fibroids in some cases, but is not a cure. The fibroids return promptly when the medicine is stopped. Shrinking the fibroids might allow minor rather than major surgery to be performed. (See surgical methods listed.) GnRh agonists are taken for a few months, but not more than six, because their side effects mimic the menopause.

There are two basic surgical methods:

Myomectomy – The fibroids are removed, but the uterus is not. The operation may be performed from inside the uterus, using an instrument called a hysteroscope. Alternatively, fibroids can be removed through a small incision in the abdomen, using an instrument called a laparoscope, or through a larger incision in the abdomen during an operation called a laparotomy.

Hysterectomy – Surgery that removes the uterus and the fibroids with it. Depending on the size of the fibroids, this can be done:

- Vaginally
- Through abdominal surgery

A hysterectomy is recommended when the fibroid is very large or when there is severe bleeding that can't be stopped by other treatments. A hysterectomy leaves a women sterile and is the only certain way, according to many experts, to get rid of fibroids. Myomectomy methods may allow fibroids to grow back. The more fibroids there are to begin with, the greater the chance they will grow back.

Questions to Ask

Do you have severe abdominal pain? **YES**

NO

Do you have any of these:
- Heavy menstrual bleeding (do you saturate a pad or tampon in less than an hour)
- Bleeding between periods or after intercourse **YES**
- Bleeding after the menopause
- Anaemia (noted by paleness, weakness, fatigue)

NO

Do you have pain:
- During sexual intercourse
- With your menstrual periods **YES**
- In the lower back, not caused by strain or any other condition

NO

Do you urinate frequently or feel pressure on your bladder or rectum? **YES**

NO

Self-Care and Preventive Procedures

- Maintain a healthy body weight. The more body fat you have, the more oestrogen your body is likely to produce, which enhances fibroid growth.
- Exercise regularly. This may reduce your body's fat and oestrogen levels.
- Eat a diet low in fat.

MENOPAUSE

The menopause is when a woman's menstrual periods stop altogether. It signals the end of fertility. A woman is said to have gone through the menopause when her menstrual periods have stopped for an entire year. 'The change', as menopause is often called, generally occurs between the ages of 45 and 55. It can, though, take place as early as 35 or as late as 65. It can also result from the surgical removal of both ovaries. The physical and emotional signs and symptoms that go with 'the change' usually span one to two years or more (perimenopause). They vary from woman to woman. The changes, themselves, are a result of a number of factors. These include hormone changes such as oestrogen decline, the aging process itself and stress.

Physical signs and symptoms associated with menopause are:
- Hot flushes are sudden waves of heat that can start in the waist or chest and work their way to the neck and face and

147

sometimes the rest of the body. They are more common in the evening and during hot weather. They can occur as often as every 90 minutes. Each one can last from 15 seconds to 30 minutes — five minutes is average. Seventy-five to 80 per cent of women going through the menopause experience hot flushes, some being more bothered by them than others. Sometimes heart palpitations accompany hot flushes.

- Irregular periods vary and can include:
  - Periods that get shorter and lighter for two or more years
  - Periods that stop for a few months and then start up again and are more widely spaced
  - Periods that bring heavy bleeding, and/or the passage of many or large blood clots. (This can lead to anaemia.)
- Vaginal dryness results from hormonal changes. The vaginal wall also becomes thinner. This drying and thinning can make sexual intercourse painful or uncomfortable and lead to irritation and increased risk of infection.
- Loss of bladder tone which can result in stress incontinence (leaking of urine when you cough, sneeze or exercise)
- Headaches, dizziness
- Skin and hair changes. Skin is more likely to wrinkle, and there may be a growth of facial hair but a thinning of hair in the temple region.
- Breast tenderness
- Bloating in the upper abdomen
- Loss of some strength and tone of muscles
- Bones become more brittle, increasing the risk of osteoporosis

- Increased risk of heart attack when oestrogen levels drop

Emotional changes associated with the menopause are:
- Irritability
- Mood changes
- Lack of concentration, difficulty with memory
- Tension, anxiety, depression
- Insomnia (may result from hot flushes that interrupt sleep)

Treatment for the symptoms of the menopause varies from woman to woman. If symptoms cause little or no distress, medical treatment is not needed. The Self-Care Procedures listed may be all that is required. Hormone replacement therapy (HRT) can reduce many of the symptoms of the menopause. It also offers significant protection against osteoporosis and heart disease. Each woman should discuss the benefits and risks of HRT with her doctor. (See 'Osteoporosis' on page 206 and 'Chest Pain' on page 81.)

Medication to treat depression and/or anxiety may be warranted in some women. Also, some medicines can help with hot flushes.

Questions to Ask

Do you have any of these:
- Pain during intercourse
- Pain or a burning sensation when passing urine
- Thick, white or coloured vaginal discharge
- Fever, chills

YES

NO

Do you have heavy bleeding with your periods or pass many or large blood clots which leaves you pale and very tired?

YES

NO

Have you begun having menstrual periods again after a gap of six months?

YES

NO

Are hot flushes severe, frequent or persistent enough to interfere with normal activities?

YES

NO

flowchart continued in next column

Do you have risk factors for osteoporosis:
- Family history of osteoporosis
- Small bone frame
- Thin
- Fair skin
- Menopause before age 48, whether natural or caused by treatment such as surgery, radiotherapy or chemotherapy
- Lack of calcium in diet
- Lack of weight-bearing exercise
- Alcohol abuse
- Hyperthyroidism
- Use of steroid drugs

YES

NO

If you're taking hormone replacement therapy, do you have any of the following:
- Side effects
- Return of menopausal symptoms

YES

NO

Self-Care Procedures

To reduce the discomfort of hot flushes, try these tactics:
- Wear lightweight clothes made of natural fibres.

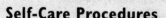

- Limit or avoid beverages that contain caffeine or alcohol.
- Avoid rich and spicy foods and heavy meals.
- Take 400 international units (I.U.) of vitamin E daily. (Consult your doctor first, though.)
- Have cool drinks, especially water, when you feel a hot flush coming on and before and after exercising. Avoid hot drinks.
- Keep cool. Open a window. Lower the thermostat when the heat is on. Use air-conditioning and/or fans. Carry a small fan with you (hand- or battery-operated).
- Try to relax when you get a hot flush. Getting stressed over one only makes it worse.
- Use relaxation techniques such as meditation, biofeedback or yoga.

If you suffer from night sweats (hot flushes that occur as you sleep):
- Wear loose-fitting cotton nightwear. Have changes of nightwear ready.
- Sleep with only a top sheet, not blankets.
- Keep the room cool.

To deal with vaginal dryness and painful intercourse:
- Don't use deodorant soaps or scented products in the vaginal area.
- Use a water-soluble lubricant (e.g., K-Y Jelly and Replens) to facilitate penetration during intercourse. Avoid oils or petroleum-based products. They encourage infection.
- Ask your doctor about intravaginal oestrogen cream.
- Remain sexually active. Having sex often may lessen the chance of having the vagina constrict and helps keep natural lubrication and maintains pelvic muscle tone. (This includes reaching orgasm with a partner or alone.)
- Drink plenty of water daily for healthy vaginal tissues.

Avoid using antihistamines unless truly necessary. They dry mucous membranes in the body.

To deal with emotional symptoms:
- Exercise regularly. This will help maintain your body's hormonal balance.
- Talk to other women who have gone through or are going through menopause. You can help each other cope with emotional symptoms.
- Avoid stressful situations as much as possible.
- Use relaxation techniques (e.g., meditation, yoga, listening to soft music, massages).
- Eat healthy. Check with your doctor about taking vitamin/mineral supplements.

PERIOD PAIN

Most women experience painful menstrual periods (dysmenorrhoea) at some time in their lives. The pain can be very mild or can be severe enough to leave a woman unable to carry out her normal activities for the first one to three days of her period. The pain may also differ from month to month, or from year to year. Cramping abdominal pains may be accompanied by backache, fatigue, vomiting, diarrhoea and headaches. The discomfort can be made worse by premenstrual bloating (water retention).

There are two types of dysmenorrhoea: primary and secondary. The primary form usually occurs in females who have just begun to menstruate. This form may disappear or become less severe after a woman reaches her mid-20s or gives birth. The cause of menstrual cramps is thought to be related to hormone-like substances called prostaglandins. These are chemicals that occur naturally in the body. Certain prostaglandins cause muscles in the uterus to go into spasm.

Dysmenorrhoea occurs much less often in women who do not ovulate. For this reason, oral contraceptives reduce painful periods in 70 to 80 per cent of women who take them. When the pill is stopped, women usually experience the same level of pain as before they took it.

Secondary dysmenorrhoea refers to period pain that is due to other disorders of the reproductive system, such as fibroids, endometriosis, ovarian cysts and, rarely, cancer. Having an intrauterine device (IUD), especially if you've never been pregnant, can also cause period pain. This problem does not occur with progesterone IUDs, which gradually release a small amount of progesterone into the uterus that reduces pain and lightens menstrual flow.

Questions to Ask

Have your menstrual periods been especially painful since having an intrauterine contraceptive device (IUD) inserted? **YES**

NO

Do you have any signs of infection such as fever and foul-smelling vaginal discharge or do you have black stools or blood in the stools? **YES**

NO

Do you have a heavier than usual blood flow and/or a period that is late by one or more weeks (for women who are still capable of bearing children)? **YES**

NO

Is the pain extreme or have you had pain-free periods for years but are now having severe cramps? **YES**

NO

Does cramping continue even after your period is over? **YES**

NO

Self-Care Procedures

To relieve menstrual cramps:

- Take aspirin or ibuprofen as directed to relieve pain and inhibit the release of prostaglandins. Paracetamol will help with pain, but not with prostaglandins. Know that most over-the-counter menstrual discomfort products contain paracetamol and not a pain reliever that also inhibits prostaglandins. Read labels. *Note: Do not give aspirin, or any medication containing salicylates, to anyone under 12 years of age, unless directed by a doctor, due to its association with Reye's syndrome, a potentially fatal condition.*
- Drink a hot cup of tea, camomile tea or mint tea.
- Whenever possible, lie on your back, supporting your knees with a pillow.
- Hold a wrapped hot-water bottle on your abdomen or lower back.
- Take a warm bath.
- Gently massage your abdomen.
- Do mild exercises such as stretching, walking or biking. Exercise may improve blood flow and reduce pelvic pain.
- Unless you have reasons to avoid alcohol, have a glass of wine or other alcoholic drink. Alcohol slows down uterine contractions.
- Get plenty of rest and avoid stressful situations as your period approaches.
- For birth control, consider using the Pill, because it blocks the production of prostaglandins, or ask your doctor about a progesterone IUD.

If you still feel pain after using Self-Care Procedures, call your doctor.

OVARIAN CYSTS

The ovaries are two plum-sized organs on either side of the uterus. They produce eggs and female hormones (oestrogen, progesterone and others). Growths called cysts can form in, on or near the ovaries. Rarely cancerous, cysts are sacs filled with fluid or semi-solid material. Ovarian cysts are commonly found in women in their reproductive years. Taking hormones does not cause cysts.

Women more likely to get ovarian cysts are:

- Between the ages of 20 and 35
- Those who have endometriosis or pelvic inflammatory disease (PID)

Signs and Symptoms

Most of the time, ovarian cysts are harmless and cause no symptoms. When symptoms do occur, they include:

- A feeling of fullness or swelling of the abdomen
- Weight gain
- A dull constant ache on either or both sides of the pelvis
- Pain during intercourse
- Delayed, irregular or painful menstrual periods
- Increased facial hair
- Sharp, severe abdominal pain, fever, and/or vomiting. This may be caused by a bleeding cyst or one that breaks or twists.

Ovarian cysts are of three basic types:

Functional cysts – This is the most common type. These cysts are related to variations in the normal function of the ovaries. They can last four to six weeks. Rarely do they secrete hormones.

Follicular and corpus luteum cysts – A follicular cyst is one in which the egg-making follicle of the ovary enlarges and fills with fluid. A corpus luteum cyst is a yellow mass of tissue that forms from the follicle after ovulation. These types of cysts come and go each month and are associated with normal ovarian function.

Abnormal cysts or neoplastic cysts – These result from abnormal cell growth. They are usually benign but in rare cases can be cancerous. Abnormal cysts require treatment by your doctor. Types of abnormal cysts include:

• Serous cysts – which contain fluid and are usually benign.
• Mucous cysts – which contain a mucus-like substance (mucus cysts) and are also usually benign.
  Other rarer types include:
• Dermoid cysts – which consist of a growth filled with various types of tissue such as fatty material, hair, teeth, bits of bone and cartilage.
• Polycystic ovaries – caused by a build-up of multiple small cysts which cause hormonal imbalances that can result in irregular periods, body hair growth and infertility.

Detection

You can find out if you have ovarian cysts through:

• A pelvic examination, in which your doctor can feel the size of your ovaries and discover abnormalities
• An ultrasound, in which sound waves create pictures of internal organs through a device placed on your abdomen or a probe inserted inside your vagina
• A laparoscopy, a minor surgical procedure which allows your doctor to see the structures inside your abdomen

Treatment

Treatment for ovarian cysts will depend on:

• Size and type of cyst(s)
• Age and whether you are in your reproductive years or have reached the menopause
• Desire to have children
• General health
• Severity of symptoms

Some cysts may disappear without any treatment within one to two months. For others, hormone therapy with oral contraceptives may be tried to suppress the cyst(s). If a cyst does not respond to this treatment, surgery may be needed to remove the cyst. If a cyst is found early, the surgery may not have to be extensive and the cyst may be removed leaving the ovary. Sometimes the ovary needs to be removed and surgery may include removal of the fallopian tube and uterus as well.

Questions to Ask

Do you have severe abdominal pain, fever and vomiting? **YES**

NO

Do you have any of the following that are not due to other known reasons:
- Abdominal fullness or swelling
- Delayed, irregular or painful menstrual periods
- Pain during intercourse
- Dull and constant ache on either or both sides of your pelvis

YES

NO

Self-Care and Preventive Procedures

- Reduce caffeine intake.
- Have regular pelvic examinations according to your doctor's recommendations.
- Take paracetamol, aspirin and ibuprofen for minor pain. *Note: Do not give aspirin, or any medication containing salicylates, to children under 12 years of age, unless directed by a doctor, due to its association with Reye's syndrome, a potentially fatal condition.*

PREMENSTRUAL SYNDROME (PMS)

Four out of 10 menstruating women suffer from premenstrual syndrome (PMS), also known as premenstrual tension (PMT). A syndrome is a group of signs and symptoms that indicate a disorder. There have been as many as 150 symptoms associated with PMS. The most common ones are:
- Irritability
- Anxiety
- Depression
- Headache
- Bloating
- Fatigue
- Feelings of hostility and anger
- Food cravings (especially for chocolate, sweet and salty foods)

The exact cause or causes of PMS are not known; however, there are many theories. One points to low levels of the hormone progesterone. Others link it to nutritional or chemical deficiencies. One thing is certain though, to be classified as PMS, symptoms must occur between ovulation and menstruation – i.e., appear anytime within the two weeks before the menstrual period, and disappear shortly after the period begins. (PMS is thought to cease with the menopause.)

For some women, symptoms are slight and may last only a few days before menstruation. For others, they can be severe and last the whole two weeks before every period. Also worth noting is that other disorders women experience (e.g., arthritis and clinical depression) may be worse during this same premenstrual period.

PMS is often confused with depression. An evaluation by your doctor can help with a correct diagnosis.

Treatments for PMS may include:

- Medical management with medicines such as:
  - The prescribed hormone proges-terone (suppositories or an oral form)
  - Water pills (diuretics)
- Dietary changes such as:
  - Eating five to six light meals instead of three large ones; not skipping meals
  - Avoiding caffeine and alcohol
  - Avoiding sweets
  - Limiting salt and fat
  - Vitamin supplements, especially B_6
  - Adequate intake of calcium and magnesium
- Lifestyle changes such as: regular exercise that includes 20 minutes of aerobic exercise (e.g., walking or aerobic dance) at least three times a week
- Limiting and learning to deal with stress

Questions to Ask

Are the symptoms of PMS (anxiety, depression, anger that leads to aggression, etc.) making you feel suicidal? YES

NO

flowchart continued in next column

Do PMS symptoms make you feel out of control and unable to live your daily life? YES

NO

Do you still have PMS symptoms after your period starts? YES

NO

Have you tried the Self-Care Procedures listed and you still don't feel better? YES

NO

Self-Care Procedures

- Exercise three times a week for 20 minutes. Swimming, walking and bicycling all relax your muscles.
- Eat five to six small meals a day instead of three large ones.
- Limit salt, fat and sugar. Choose healthy food options and avoid junk foods.
- If you need to satisfy a food craving, do so in moderation. For example, if you crave chocolate, eat only a small bar. If you crave salt, eat only a small packet of crisps.
- Avoid caffeine, alcohol and cigarettes for two weeks before your period is due.

- The supplements listed here seem to help some women. Ask your doctor if you should take them and in what amounts:
  Vitamin B_6
  Vitamin E
- Evening primrose oil
  Calcium
  Magnesium
  L-tyrosine, an amino acid
- Take naps if PMS keeps you up at night.
- Learn to relax. Try deep breathing, meditation, yoga or a hot bath.
- Try to avoid stress when you have PMS.

TOXIC SHOCK SYNDROME

Toxic shock syndrome (TSS) is a potentially fatal disease caused by bacteria. It is a form of blood poisoning that results when poisons (toxins) are released by certain bacteria. It can result from wounds or infection in the throat, lungs, skin or bone. It has also occurred in a number of women who were using superabsorbent tampons. These tampons (no longer on sale in the UK) trapped the bacteria and provided a breeding ground for them, especially when left in place for a long time. In rare cases, failure to remove an ordinary tampon for a long time at the end of a period can also result in TSS. Though not common, TSS can also occur in people after surgery, including women who have had caesarean sections. Symptoms come on fast and are often severe:

- High, sudden fever
- Muscle aches
- Vomiting
- Diarrhoea
- Sunburn-like rash, including peeling skin on hands and feet
- Rapid pulse
- Extreme fatigue and weakness
- Sore throat
- Dizziness
- Fainting
- Drop in blood pressure

Prevention

Take the following precautions to prevent TSS:
- Change tampons and sanitary towels at least every four to six hours.

Questions to Ask

Are any of the symptoms of toxic shock syndrome (see list) present? YES

NO

THRUSH (CANDIDIASIS)

Thrush, also known as candidiasis, is the most common type of vaginal infection. It results from the overgrowth of *Candida albicans*, a type of yeast that is normally present in harmless amounts in the vagina, the digestive tract and the mouth. Some women rarely get thrush; others get it regularly. It may be triggered by:

- Hormonal changes that come with pregnancy or before the monthly periods
- Taking hormones, including birth control pills
- Taking antibiotics, especially 'broad-spectrum' ones
- Taking steroid drugs such as prednisone
- Having raised blood sugar, such as occurs in uncontrolled diabetes
- Vaginal intercourse, especially with inadequate lubrication

Symptoms can range from mild to severe. They include:

- Itching, irritation and redness around the external genitalia
- A thick, white discharge that looks like cottage cheese. (It may smell like yeast.)
- Burning and/or pain when you urinate or have sex

- Use unscented tampons or sanitary towels and change tampons and sanitary towels frequently.
- Don't use bath oils, bubble baths, feminine hygiene sprays, and perfumed or deodorant soaps.
- Don't sit around in a wet bathing costume.
- Shower after you swim in a pool to remove the chlorine from your skin. Dry the vaginal area thoroughly.
- If you tend to get thrush whenever you take an antibiotic, ask your doctor to prescribe a vaginal antifungal agent as well, or use an over-the-counter one.
- Eat well. Include foods such as yogurt that contains live cultures of lactobacillus acidophilus.
- Make sure your partner is checked for infection and treated, especially if you get recurring infections. This will avoid reinfection.
- Get plenty of rest for your body to fight infections.

Prevention

- Practise good hygiene. Wash regularly but don't use soap in the genital area. Dry area thoroughly after you shower or bathe.
- Wipe from front to back after using the toilet.
- Wear all-cotton panties.
- Don't wear slacks and shorts that are tight in the crutch and thighs, or other tight-fitting clothing such as panty girdles.
- Change underwear and work-out clothes immediately after exercising.

Treatment

Treatment for thrush consists mostly of vaginal creams or suppositories that get rid of the yeast overgrowth. These can be over-the-counter ones (ask your pharmacist) or ones prescribed by your doctor.

First and foremost, though, is the need to make sure you have the problem correctly diagnosed. A burning sensation could be a symptom of a urinary tract infection caused by bacteria that requires an antibiotic. Antibiotics do not cure a yeast infection; they only make it worse. Check with your doctor if you are not sure that your problem is thrush, especially if this is the first time you have symptoms of it and if the infection you treat comes back within two months or does not respond to treatment at all.

Chronic thrush can be one of the first signs of diabetes or of sexually transmitted diseases in women.

directed. Women who have had thrush whenever they have taken antibiotics in the past should use these preparations during the period of antibiotic treatment.
- Eat yogurt and other foods that contain live cultures of lactobacillus acidophilus several times daily (especially when taking an antibiotic).

Questions to Ask

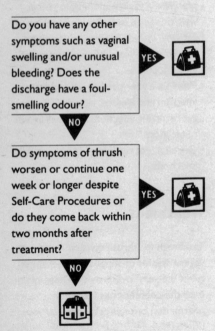

Do you have any other symptoms such as vaginal swelling and/or unusual bleeding? Does the discharge have a foul-smelling odour?

YES

NO

Do symptoms of thrush worsen or continue one week or longer despite Self-Care Procedures or do they come back within two months after treatment?

YES

NO

Self-Care Procedures

To get rid of thrush, try the following:
- Use an over-the-counter treatment, in the form of a cream or suppositories, as

CHAPTER 10
MEN'S HEALTH

ENLARGED PROSTATE

The prostate gland is walnut-shaped and produces seminal fluid. Located below a man's bladder, it actually surrounds a portion of the bladder and the beginning of the urethra (tube that carries urine away from the bladder). If they live long enough, most men will eventually suffer from an enlarged prostate gland – a condition called benign prostatic hypertrophy (BPH).

An enlarged prostate is troublesome but is usually not cancerous or life-threatening. The symptoms are:

• Increased urgency to urinate
• Frequent urination, especially during the night
• Delay in onset of urine flow
• Diminished or slow stream of urine flow
• Incomplete emptying of the bladder.

These symptoms indicate that the prostate gland has enlarged enough partially to obstruct the flow of urine. Sometimes BPH causes a urinary tract infection (UTI). Over time, a few men might have bladder or kidney problems or both.

Your doctor can diagnose BPH using a number of methods. These include:

• An examination that includes asking questions about your current symptoms and past medical problems, rectal examination of the prostate gland, a check of your urine for signs of infection and a blood test to determine if the prostate has affected your kidneys.
• Tests that measure urine flow, the amount of urine left in your bladder after you urinate and the pressure in your bladder as you urinate.
• A blood test called a prostate-specific antigen (PSA) test, which can help detect prostate cancer. Not all doctors agree that being tested for PSA levels lowers a person's chance of dying from prostate cancer. The PSA test is not always accurate either. You should discuss this test with your doctor.
• Other tests such as X-rays, cystoscopy (in which the doctor directly views the prostate and the lining of the bladder) and an ultrasound (sound wave pictures) of the prostate, kidneys or bladder. Many men do not need these tests.

Treatment for BPH varies depending on symptoms. Discuss the benefits and possible problems with your doctor for each treatment option. Treatment options include:

Watchful waiting – Regular follow-up visits to the doctor to see if your BPH is causing problems or getting worse.

Medications – There are two types:
• Alpha blockers which help relax muscles in the prostate.

- Finasteride, which causes the prostate to shrink.

These medications may not reduce need for surgery but they may delay it. They also can have side effects, so you should see your doctor for monitoring.

Balloon dilatation – a day-case surgical procedure performed in hospital. A balloon-tipped catheter is inserted into the penis, through the urethra and into the bladder. The balloon is inflated to stretch the urethra in order to allow urine to flow more easily.

Surgery – This may be:
- Transurethral resection of the prostate (TURP), which is the most common type. The part of the prostate around the urethra is removed from inside the urethra. There is no scar. The operation relieves symptoms by reducing pressure on the urethra and is a proven way to treat BPH effectively.
- Open prostatectomy, which may be used if the prostate is very large. An incision is made in the lower abdomen to remove part of the inside of the prostate.

Prostate surgery can result in problems such as impotence and/or incontinence. Most men, however, who undergo surgery have no major problems. Nonetheless, it is important to discuss the benefits and risks of these procedures with your doctor.

Questions to Ask

Do you have one or more of these problems:
- A feeling that you have to urinate right away, or the need to urinate often, especially at night
- A feeling that you can't empty your bladder completely
- A feeling of hesitancy or delay, or straining to urinate
- A weak or interrupted urinary flow

 YES

NO

Do you have one or more of these symptoms of an infection that may result from BPH:
- Burning, frequent or painful urination
- Pain in the lower back, groin or testicles
- Pain in or near the penis
- Pain on ejaculation
- Discharge from the penis (blood or pus)
- Fever and/or chills

 YES

NO

Self-Care Procedures

- Remain sexually active.
- Take hot baths.
- Avoid dampness and cold temperatures.
- Do not let the bladder get too full. Urinate as soon as the urge arises. Relax when you urinate.
- When you take long trips, make frequent stops to urinate. Keep a container in the car that you can urinate in when you can't get to a toilet in time.
- Limit coffee, tea, alcohol and spicy foods.
- Drink eight or more glasses of water every day, but don't drink liquids too close to bedtime.
- Reduce stress.
- Don't smoke.
- Avoid over-the-counter antihistamines.

JOCK ITCH

Jock itch is typified by redness, itching and scaliness in the groin and thigh area, and is usually caused by a fungus infection. It can also result from a bacterial infection or be a reaction to chemicals in clothing, irritating garments or medicines.

Jock itch gets its name because an athletic support worn during exercise, which is subsequently stored in a dark, poorly ventilated locker, then perhaps worn again without being laundered, provides the ideal environment for the fungi to thrive. (Under similar conditions, women's clothing can develop this problem, too.)

Questions to Ask

Do symptoms of jock itch persist longer than two weeks despite Self-Care Procedures? **YES**

NO

Self-Care Procedures

To relieve jock itch and prevent future attacks:

- Don't wear tight, close-fitting clothing. Boxer shorts are recommended for men.
- Change underwear frequently, especially after work, if you have a job that leaves you hot and sweaty.
- Bathe or shower immediately after exercising.
- Apply talc or other powder to the groin area to help keep it dry.
- Don't store damp clothing in a locker or gym bag. Wash work-out clothes after each use.
- Sleep in the nude.
- Avoid antibacterial (deodorant) soaps.

An over-the-counter antifungal cream, powder or lotion should be used (ask your pharmacist). It needs to be continued for at least two weeks to avoid recurrence of the problem.

TESTICULAR CANCER AND TESTICULAR SELF-EXAMINATION

Cancer of the testicles accounts for only about 1 per cent of all cancers in men. It is, though, the most common type of cancer in males aged 20 to 40, but can occur any time after about age 15. Often only one testicle is affected.

The cause of testicular cancer is not known. However, there are known risk factors, such as:

- Uncorrected undescended testicles in infant and young boys. (Parents should see that their infant boys are checked at birth for undescended testicles.)
- A family history of testicular cancer
- Having an identical twin with testicular cancer.

Signs and Symptoms

In the early stages, testicular cancer may have no symptoms. When there are symptoms, they include:

- Small, painless lump in a testicle
- Enlarged testicle
- Feeling of heaviness in the testicle or groin
- Pain in the testicle
- A change in the way the testicle feels
- Enlarged male breasts and nipples
- Blood or fluid suddenly accumulating in the scrotum.

Testicular cancer is curable 90 to 95 per cent of cases if found and treated early. The testicle is surgically removed.

Further treatment may include:
- Chemotherapy
- Radiotherapy
- Surgically removing nearby lymph nodes if necessary.

Questions to Ask

Do you have severe testicular pain? **YES**

NO

Can any lumps, enlargement, swelling or change in consistency be felt in the scrotum? **YES**

NO

Is there any sense of heaviness or pain? **YES**

NO

Is there an enlargement of the breasts and nipples or a sudden feeling of puffiness in the scrotum? **YES**

NO

Testicular Self-Examination

The testicles are located behind the penis and contained within the scrotum. They should be about the same size and feel smooth, rubbery and egg-shaped. The left one sometimes hangs lower than the right.

Regular self-examination of the testicles is recommended from puberty onwards. Examination is best performed when the scrotum is relaxed, after a warm bath or shower. This will also allow the testicles to drop down.

How to examine the testicles:

- Examine each testicle gently with both hands. The index and middle fingers should be placed underneath the testicle while the thumbs are placed on the top. Roll the testicle gently between the thumbs and fingers. One testicle may be larger than the other. This is normal.

- The epididymis is a cord-like structure on the top and back of the testicle that stores and transports the sperm. Do not confuse the epididymis with an abnormal lump.

- Feel for any abnormal lumps (about the size of a pea) on the front or the side of the testicle. These lumps are usually painless.

If you do find a lump, you should contact your doctor right away. The lump may be due to an infection, and a doctor can decide the proper treatment. If the lump is not due to an infection, it is likely to be cancer. Remember, though, that testicular cancer is highly curable, especially when detected and treated early. Testicular cancer almost always occurs in only one testicle, and the other testicle is all that is needed for full sexual function.

CHAPTER 11
SEXUALLY TRANSMITTED DISEASES (STDs)

Infections that pass from one person to another during sexual contact are known as sexually transmitted diseases (STDs). Sexual contact is defined as vaginal, anal or oral sex.

Sexually transmitted diseases include chlamydia, gonorrhoea, syphilis, genital herpes and trichomoniasis. Acquired immune deficiency syndrome (AIDS) is often classified as a sexually transmitted disease, but it can be passed through means other than sexual contact. So, though mentioned at times, it is not defined here. (See page 180 for information on AIDS.) Note, though, that the Self-Care Prevention Procedures listed can help prevent sexually acquired infection with human immunodeficiency virus (HIV) (see page 181).

BASIC FACTS ABOUT STDS

Signs and symptoms

STDs are transmitted through intimate sexual contact. Each STD has its own set of symptoms, but a discharge from the penis or vagina, pain when urinating (in males), and open sores or blisters in the genital area are typical of most STDs. Unfortunately, early stages of STDs often have no detectable symptoms. In

addition, you can also have more than one STD at the same time. Gonorrhoea and chlamydia, for example, are often acquired at the same time.

Treatment

If you suspect you have an STD, see a doctor as soon as possible. Your sexual partner(s) should also be contacted and treated.

Depending on the infection, STDs can cause serious, long-term problems like birth defects, infertility, diseases of the brain or, in the case of AIDS, death.

Some STDs can be treated and cured with antibiotics. For others, such as AIDS, there is no cure. Prevention is the only treatment.

At present, no vaccines exist to prevent STDs. And once you've had an STD, you can get it again. You can't develop an immunity once you've been exposed.

(Note: Medical treatment, not self-care treatment, is necessary for sexually transmitted diseases. One exception is genital herpes for which many self-care remedies can help alleviate the discomfort that occurs with recurrent attacks. Self-Care Prevention Procedures, however, should be followed to lower the risk of contracting STDs. [See page 170.])

CHLAMYDIA

Chlamydia is the most common sexually transmitted disease (STD) in the UK. It is thought to affect more men and women than syphilis, gonorrhoea and genital herpes combined. In fact, the chances are that people who have had these other STDs are playing host to chlamydia as well. Chlamydia can also accelerate the appearance of AIDS symptoms for persons infected with HIV.

Symptoms of chlamydia in men include burning or discomfort when urinating, a whitish discharge from the tip of the penis, and pain in the scrotum. In women, symptoms include slight yellowish-green vaginal discharge, vaginal irritation, a frequent need to urinate, and pain when urinating. There can also be chronic abdominal pain and bleeding between menstrual periods.

These symptoms can, however, be so mild that they often go unnoticed. It is estimated that 75 per cent of women and 25 per cent of men who have chlamydia have no symptoms until complications set in. If symptoms do appear, they usually do so two to four weeks after being infected.

The only sure way to know whether or not you have chlamydia is to be tested. Tests are performed at hospital genito-urinary clinics.

Anyone who has chlamydia should be treated with oral antibiotics (e.g., tetracycline or erythromycin) for two to three weeks. Doctors will treat the infected sexual partner even if he or she doesn't show any symptoms. Sex should be avoided until treatment is completed in both the person affected and in his or her sex partners. If left untreated, chlamydia can cause a variety of serious problems, including infection and inflammation of the prostate and surrounding structures in men and pelvic inflammatory disease (PID) and infertility in women. Infants born to mothers who have chlamydia at the time of delivery are likely to develop pneumonia or serious eye infections in the first few months of life as well as permanent lung damage later on.

Questions to Ask

For men: Do you have these problems?
- A whitish discharge from the penis, burning or discomfort when urinating, pain and swelling in the scrotum?

YES

NO

For women: Do you have these problems?
- A yellowish-green vaginal discharge
- Frequent need to urinate
- Chronic abdominal pain
- Bleeding between menstrual periods

YES

NO

flowchart continued on next page

| Does your sexual partner have or do you suspect he or she might have a sexually transmitted disease? Does he or she have multiple sex partners? | **YES** ▶ | |

 NO

| Do you want to rule out the presence of chlamydia because you are considering a new sexual relationship, planning to get married or pregnant, or for any other reason? | **YES** ▶ | |

 NO

GENITAL HERPES

Herpes simplex virus II (HSVII) is spread by direct skin-to-skin contact from the site of infection to the contact site. Once you are infected, the virus remains with you forever. It causes symptoms, though, only during flare-ups.

Symptoms include sores with blisters on the genital area and anus, and sometimes on the thighs and buttocks. After a few days, the blisters break open and leave painful, shallow ulcers which can last from five days to three weeks. If infected for the first time, you may experience flu-like symptoms such as swollen glands, fever and body aches, but subsequent attacks are almost always much milder. These attacks may be triggered by emotional stress, fatigue, menstruation, other illnesses or even by vigorous sexual intercourse. Itching, irritation and tingling in the genital area may occur one to two days before the outbreak of the blisters or sores. (This period is called the prodrome.) Genital herpes is contagious after blisters appear and up to a week or two after they have disappeared. If a pregnant woman has an outbreak of genital herpes when her baby is due, a caesarean section may need to be performed so the baby does not get infected during delivery.

No cure exists for genital herpes. Treatment includes the drug acyclovir (Zovirax), which is available in oral and topical forms, and self-help measures to treat herpes symptoms. (See Self-Care Procedures for Genital Herpes.) Medical care is especially helpful during the first attack of genital herpes. Self-help remedies may be all that is necessary during recurrent episodes.

In some people herpes-like sores and blisters can be a side effect of taking certain prescription medicine. One example is sulpha drugs which are sometimes used to treat urinary tract infections. Consult your doctor if you suspect this.

Questions to Ask

Do you have sores and/or painful blisters on the genital area, anus or tongue, and is this the first time you have had this? Do you have a mild fever, headache, general muscle ache and a general feeling of illness? **YES**

NO

Did these sores appear only after taking a recently prescribed medicine? **YES**

NO

For people who have already been diagnosed as having genital herpes: Do you have severe pain and blistering and/or frequent attacks? **YES**

NO

For pregnant women: Are these sores present and are you close to your delivery date? **YES**

NO

Have you had sexual relations with someone who had sores or blisters on their genital area, anus or tongue or had genital itching, irritation and tingling? **YES**

NO

Self-Care Procedures for Genital Herpes

- Bathe the affected genital area twice a day with mild soap and water. Gently pat dry with a towel or use a hair dryer set on warm.
- Apply ice packs to the genital area for five to 10 minutes. This may help relieve itching and inflammation.
- Wear loose-fitting pants or skirts. Avoid wearing panty hose and tight-fitting clothing. These could irritate the inflamed area. Wear cotton, not nylon underwear.
- Squirt tepid water over the genital area while urinating. This may help decrease the pain.
- Take a mild pain reliever such as aspirin, paracetamol or ibuprofen. *Note: Do not give aspirin, or any medication containing salicylates, to children under 12 years of age, unless directed by a doctor, due to its association with Reye's syndrome, a potentially fatal condition.*
- Use an antiviral drug such as acyclovir (Zovirax), which your doctor may prescribe for you.
- To avoid spreading the virus to your eyes, don't touch your eyes during an outbreak.
  - Avoid sexual intercourse:
    - At the first sign of a herpes outbreak. (This may be evident by the feeling of tingling and itching in the genital area and takes place before blisters are noticeable.) Note, though, that herpes can be contracted even though there are no visible blisters, because blisters

may be present on the female's cervix or inside the male's urethra.

- When blisters are present
- One to two weeks after blisters have disappeared

GONORRHOEA

Gonorrhoea is one of the most common infectious diseases in the world. Often called 'the clap' or 'a dose', it is caused by specific bacterium that is transmitted during vaginal, oral or anal sex. A newborn baby can also get gonorrhoea during birth if its mother is infected. Gonorrhoea can be symptom-free. In fact, about 60 to 80 per cent of infected women have no symptoms.

The signs of gonorrhoea can, however, show up within two to 10 days after sexual contact with an infected person. In men, symptoms include pain at the tip of the penis, pain and burning during urination and a thick, yellow, cloudy penile discharge that gradually increases. In women, symptoms include mild itching and burning around the vagina, a thick yellowish-green vaginal discharge, burning on urination and severe lower abdominal pain (usually within a week or so after a menstrual period).

If ignored, gonorrhoea can cause widespread infection and/or infertility. But gonorrhoea can be cured with injections of specific antibiotics. If you've been infected with a type of gonorrhoea that's resistant to penicillin, your doctor will have to use another medicine.

To treat gonorrhoea successfully, you should heed the following:
- Take prescribed medications.
- To avoid reinfection, be sure that your sexual partner is also treated.
- Have follow-up tests to determine if the treatment was effective.

Questions to Ask

For men: Do you have any of these problems:
- A discharge of pus from the penis
- Discomfort or pain when urinating
- Irritation and itching of the penis
- Pain during intercourse

YES

For women: Do you have any of these problems:
- Itching and burning around the vagina
- A vaginal discharge (this could be slight, cloudy or yellowish-green in colour with a foul odour)
- Burning or pain when urinating
- The need to urinate often
- Discomfort in the lower abdomen
- Abnormal bleeding from the vagina

YES

NO

flowchart continued on next page

Are you symptom-free, but may have contracted gonorrhoea or another sexually transmitted disease from someone you suspect may be infected? **YES**

NO

Do you want to rule out the presence of a sexually transmitted disease because you have had multiple sex partners and you are considering a new sexual relationship or planning to get married or pregnant? **YES**

NO

See Self-Care Preventative Procedures Listed

SYPHILIS

Syphilis is sometimes called 'pox'. Left untreated, syphilis is one of the most serious sexually transmitted diseases, leading to heart failure, blindness, insanity or death. Syphilis can progress slowly, through three stages, over a period of many years. When detected early, however, syphilis can be cured. Be alert for the following symptoms.

Primary stage

A large, painless, ulcer-like sore known as a chancre develops two to six weeks after infection and generally appears around the area of sexual contact. The chancre disappears within a few weeks.

Secondary stage

Within a month after the end of the primary stage, a widespread skin rash appears, cropping up on the palms of the hands, soles of the feet and sometimes around the mouth and nose. The rash is composed of small, red, scaling bumps that do not itch. Swollen lymph nodes, fever and flu-like symptoms may also occur. Small patches of hair may fall out of the scalp, beard, eyelashes and eyebrows.

Latent stage

Once syphilis reaches this stage, it may go unnoticed for years, quietly damaging the heart, central nervous system, muscles and various other organs and tissues. The resulting effects are often fatal.

If you've been exposed to syphilis or have its symptoms, see your doctor or go to your local hospital genito-urinary clinic. For syphilis in its early stages, treatment consists of a single injection of long-lasting penicillin. If the disease has progressed further, you will require three consecutive weekly injections. (If you're allergic to penicillin, you will receive an alternative antibiotic, taken orally for two to four weeks.) You should have a blood test three, six and 12 months after treatment to be sure the disease is completely cured.

Once treatment is complete, you're no longer contagious. But if syphilis is left untreated, you're contagious for up to one year after you first contract the infection.

Questions to Ask

Do you have a large, painless, ulcer-like sore (chancre) in the genital area, anus or mouth? **YES**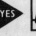

NO

Did you have such a sore two to six weeks ago that healed, but now have flu-like symptoms (fever, headache, general feeling of illness) and/or a skin rash of small, red, scaling bumps that do not itch? **YES**

NO

Are you suspicious of having contracted syphilis or another sexually transmitted disease from someone you suspect may be infected?

NO

flowchart continued in next column

Do you want to rule out the presence of syphilis or another sexually transmitted disease because you or your sex partner has had multiple sex partners and are considering a new sexual relationship, planning to get married or pregnant? **YES**

NO

See Self-Care Prevention Procedures Listed

Self-Care Prevention Procedures

• There's only one way to guarantee you'll never get a sexually transmitted disease: Never have sex.

• Limiting your sexual activity to one person your entire life is a close second, provided your partner is also monogamous and does not have a sexually transmitted disease.

• Avoid sexual contact with persons whose health and practices are not known.

• Discuss a new partner's sexual history with him or her before beginning a sexual relationship. (Be aware, though, that persons are not always honest about their sexual history.)

• Condoms can reduce the spread of sexually transmitted diseases when used properly and carefully and for every sex act. They do not eliminate the risk entirely.

- Plan ahead for safe sex. Decide what you'll say and be willing to do with a potential sex partner. Both women and men should carry condoms and insist that they be used every time they have sex.
- Using spermicidal foams, jellies, creams (especially those that contain Nonoxynol–9) and a diaphragm can offer additional protection when used with a condom. Use water-based lubricants. Don't use oil-based ones (e.g. Vaseline); they can damage condoms.
- Don't have sex while under the influence of drugs or alcohol, except in a monogamous relationship in which neither partner is infected with an STD.
- Avoid sex if either partner has signs and symptoms of a genital tract infection.
- Wash the genitals with soap and water before and after sex.
- Seek treatment for a sexually transmitted disease if you know your sex partner is infected.
- Have a check-up at a hospital genito-urinary clinic every six months if you have multiple sex partners, even if you don't have any symptoms.

CHAPTER 12
DENTAL HEALTH

ABSCESS

A tooth abscess is formed when there is inflammation and/or infection in the bone and/or the tooth's canals. This generally occurs in a tooth that has a deep cavity, a very deep filling or one that has been injured. The pain caused by a tooth abscess can be persistent, throbbing and severe. Other symptoms include fever, earache and swelling of the glands on one side of the face or neck. It can also cause a general feeling of illness, bad breath and a foul taste in the mouth.

A tooth abscess is usually treated with either root canal treatment or by extracting the tooth. A root canal is done if the dentist thinks the tooth can be saved. The infection is first removed either through a hole drilled through the top of the tooth or through an incision made in the gums at the site of the infection. These measures relieve the pain and pressure caused by a tooth abscess. An antibiotic will also be prescribed.

For the most part, tooth abscesses can be prevented with regular dental care. This includes daily brushing (with a fluoride toothpaste) and flossing and regular dental check-ups and cleaning of the teeth by your dentist.

Questions to Ask

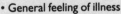

Do you have one or more of these problems as well as toothache:
- Continuous or throbbing pain
- Fever
- Earache
- Neck or jaw tenderness or swollen glands on the side where the tooth aches
- General feeling of illness
- Bad breath and/or foul taste in the mouth

YES

 NO

Does the pain come and go or only occur when you are eating or drinking? YES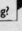

 NO

Self-Care Procedures

- To reduce pain, take aspirin, paracetamol or ibuprofen. *Note: Do not give aspirin, or any medication containing salicylates, to children under 12 years of age, unless directed by a doctor, due to its*

association with Reye's syndrome, a potentially fatal condition.
- Hold an ice pack on the jaw. This will relieve some of the pain.
- Never place a crushed aspirin on the tooth. Aspirin burns the gums and destroys tooth enamel.
- Do not drink extremely hot or cold liquids.
- Do not chew gum.
- Avoid sweets and hot and spicy foods. A liquid diet may be necessary for a day or two until the pain subsides.
- Gargle with warm salt water every hour.
- See a dentist even if the pain subsides.

BROKEN OR KNOCKED-OUT TOOTH

Your teeth are meant to last a lifetime. To protect your teeth from damage and injury, take these precautions:
- Don't chew ice, pens or pencils.
- Don't use your teeth to open paper clips or otherwise to function as tools.
- If you smoke a pipe, don't bite down on the stem.
- If you grind your teeth at night, ask your dentist if you should have a bite guard fitted to prevent tooth grinding.
- If you play contact sports such as rugby, wear a protective mouth guard.
- Always wear a seat belt when riding in a car.
- Avoid sucking on lemons or chewing aspirin or vitamin C tablets. The acid wears away tooth enamel. *Note: Do not give aspirin, or any medication containing salicylates, to children under 12 years of*

age, unless directed by a doctor, due to its association with Reye's syndrome, a potentially fatal condition.

If a tooth is accidentally knocked out, try at once to push it firmly back into the socket. Make sure it is the right way round. If you can't put the tooth back in, put it in milk and take it to the dentist immediately. Your dentist may be able to put it back in successfully. If the reimplantation can be accomplished within about half an hour, there is a possibility that the interior pulp will survive. Even up to six hours, the outer tissue of the tooth may survive and allow successful reattachment. There is little chance that the tooth can be put back in 24 hours after it has been knocked out.

Questions to Ask

Have one or more teeth been broken or knocked out? *(Note: See a dentist as soon as possible. This is a dental emergency.)* YES

NO

Self-Care Procedures

For a broken tooth:
- To reduce swelling, apply a cold compress to the area.
- Save any broken tooth fragments and take them to the dentist.

If your tooth has been knocked out:
- Rinse the tooth with clear water.
- If possible (and if you're alert), gently put it back in the socket or hold it under your tongue. Otherwise, put the tooth in a glass of milk or a wet cloth.
- If the gum is bleeding, hold a gauze pad, a clean handkerchief or a tissue tightly in place over the wound.
- Try to get to a dentist within 30 minutes of the accident.

PERIODONTAL (GUM) DISEASE

Plaque build-up, crooked teeth, illness, poorly fitting dentures, trapped food particles and certain medications can irritate or destroy your gums. With good oral hygiene, however, you can prevent periodontal (gum) disease. If caught in the early stages, gum disease is easily treated. If ignored, the gums and supporting tissues wither and your teeth may loosen and fall out.

Knowing the signs and symptoms of periodontal disease is important for early treatment. Pay attention to the following:
- Swollen red gums that bleed easily (a condition called gingivitis)
- Teeth that are exposed at the gum line (a sign that gums have pulled away from the teeth)
- Permanent teeth that are loose or separating from each other
- Bad breath and a foul taste in the mouth
- Pus around the gums and teeth
  Your dentist may be able to treat you or you may need to be referred to a

periodontist, a dentist who specializes in this area of dentistry. Material called tartar or calculus (which is calcified plaque) can form even when normal brushing and flossing are done. The dentist or dental hygienist should remove tartar at regular intervals. When periodontitis (pockets of infection and areas of weakened bone) are established, the dentist can treat the problem with surgery or with a process known as 'deep scaling'.

Questions to Ask

Are one or more of the symptoms of gum disease present:
- Swollen gums
- Gums that bleed easily
- Teeth exposed at the gum line
- Loose teeth
- Teeth separating from each other
- Pus around gums and teeth
- Bad breath and/or a foul taste in the mouth

YES

NO

Self-Care Procedures

- Make sure you brush and floss your teeth regularly.
- Use a soft, rounded bristle toothbrush (unless your dentist has told you otherwise). Ask your dentist or hygienist to show you how to brush and floss your teeth correctly.
- Eat sugary foods infrequently. When you eat sweets, do so with meals, not between meals. Finish meals with cheese because this tends to neutralize acid formation.
- Eat foods that are good sources of vitamins A and C daily. (These two vitamins promote gum health.) Vitamin A can be found in melons, broccoli, spinach, liver and dairy products fortified with vitamin A. Good vitamin C food sources include oranges, grapefruit, tomatoes, potatoes, green peppers and broccoli.

TEMPORO-MANDIBULAR JOINT SYNDROME (TMJ)

Temporo-mandibular joint syndrome (TMJ) occurs when the muscles, joints and ligaments of the jaw move out of alignment. Resulting symptoms include earaches, headaches, pain in the jaw area radiating to the face or the neck and shoulders, ringing in the ears or pain when opening and closing the mouth. These TMJ symptoms frequently mimic other conditions, so the problem is often misdiagnosed. TMJ has a number of possible causes:

- Bruxism (grinding your teeth in your sleep)
- Sleeping in a way that misaligns the jaw or creates tension in the neck
- Stress-induced muscle tension in the neck and shoulders
- Incorrect or uneven bite

TMJ may or may not require professional treatment. The condition, however, should be evaluated by a dentist. You may need to be referred to a maxillo-facial surgeon for specialist treatment. He or she may prescribe anti-inflammatory medicine, tranquilizers or muscle relaxants for a short period of time, braces to correct the bite or a bite plate to wear when sleeping. Some doctors recommend surgery to correct TMJ, but you should get more than one opinion before consenting to a surgical remedy.

Questions to Ask

 Are you unable to open or close your mouth because of severe pain? YES

NO

flowchart continued on next page

175

Do you experience one or more of the following:

- Inability to open the jaw completely
- Pain when you open your mouth widely
- Persistent symptoms of headache, earache or pain in the jaw area that is also felt in the face, neck or shoulders
- 'Clicking' or 'popping' sounds when you open your mouth and when you chew

YES

NO

Self-Care Procedures

If you have TMJ, you may be able to minimize symptoms in the following ways:

- Don't chew gum.
- Try not to open your jaw wide (including yawning or taking big bites out of large sandwiches or other difficult-to-eat foods).
- Massage the jaw area several times a day, first with your mouth open, then with your mouth closed.
- To help reduce muscle spasms that can cause pain, apply moist heat to the jaw area. (A washcloth soaked in warm water makes a convenient hot compress.)
- If stress is a factor, consider biofeedback and relaxation training.

TOOTHACHES

The pain of a toothache can be felt in the tooth itself or in the region around the tooth. Most toothaches are usually the result of either a cavity or an infection beneath or around the gum of a tooth. Insufficient oxygen to the heart as experienced with angina or a heart attack can also cause pain in the jaw. Toothache is common after having corrective dental work on a tooth, but should not last longer than a week. (If it does, inform the dentist.)

Generally, toothaches can be prevented with regular visits to the dentist and daily self-care measures. Self-care includes proper daily brushing and flossing, good nutrition and using fluoridated water, toothpastes, rinses and supplements (if prescribed).

Because these may lead to a toothache if left unchecked, tell your dentist if you notice any of the following:

- Sensitivity to hot, cold or sweet foods
- Brown spots or little holes on a tooth
- A change in your bite (the way your teeth fit together)
- Loose teeth in an adult

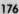

Questions to Ask

Do you have any of these problems as well as toothache:
- Gnawing pain in the lower teeth or neck
- Chest discomfort beneath the breast bone
- Pain that travels to or is felt in the shoulder or arm
- Sweating

YES

NO

Are any of the following symptoms present:
- Fever
- Red, swollen or bleeding gums
- Swollen face
- Foul breath even after thorough brushing and flossing
- Constant toothache even when sleeping at night
- Toothache only when eating or just after eating

YES

NO

Self-Care Procedures

- To reduce discomfort, take aspirin or another mild pain reliever. *Note: Do not give aspirin, or any medication containing salicylates, to children under 12 years of age, unless directed by a doctor, due to its association with Reye's syndrome, a potentially fatal condition.*
- Hold an ice pack on the jaw. This will relieve some of the pain.
- Never place a crushed aspirin on the tooth. Aspirin burns the gums and destroys tooth enamel.
- Do not drink extremely hot or cold liquids.
- Do not chew gum.
- Avoid sweets, soft drinks and hot and spicy foods. (These can irritate cavities and increase pain.) It may be best not to eat at all until you see your dentist.
- Gargle with warm salt water every hour.
- For a cavity, pack it with a piece of sterile cotton wool soaked in oil of cloves (available at chemists).
- See a dentist even if the pain subsides.

SECTION 2
MAJOR MEDICAL CONDITIONS

INTRODUCTION

Section 2 covers 30 major medical conditions. Where applicable, the discussions of the conditions includes the following:

• Information about the condition
• Signs and symptoms of the condition
• Treatment and care for the condition
• Strategies for prevention

Unlike the common health problems in Section 1, which you may be able to treat with Self-Care Procedures alone, these 30 medical conditions need a doctor's diagnosis and medical treatment from health care professionals. However, there will be things you still need to do to take care of yourself if you have any of these conditions.

CHAPTER 13
MAJOR MEDICAL CONDITIONS

AIDS

AIDS is an acronym for acquired immune deficiency syndrome. It is caused by the human immunodeficiency virus (HIV). This virus destroys the body's immune system, leaving the person unable to fight certain types of infection and cancer. The AIDS virus also attacks the central nervous system, causing mental and neurological problems.

The virus is carried in bodily fluids (semen, vaginal secretions, blood and breast milk).

Certain activities are likely to promote contracting the AIDS virus. High-risk activities include:

• Unprotected* anal, oral and/or vaginal sex except in a monogamous relationship in which neither partner is infected with HIV. Particularly high-risk situations are having sex:
  • When drunk or high on drugs
  • With multiple or casual sex partners
  • With a partner who has had multiple or casual sex partners
  • With a partner who has used drugs by injection or is bisexual
  • When you or your partner has signs and symptoms of a genital tract infection
• Sharing needles and/or other items when injecting any kind of drugs

• Pregnancy and delivery if the mother is infected with HIV. (This can put the child at risk.)
• Having blood transfusions or using blood products (e.g., factor VIII) before routine testing for HIV was introduced

* Unprotected sex means without condoms. When used correctly, every time and for every sex act condoms provide protection from HIV. Though not 100 per cent effective, they will reduce the risk.

There is some concern about the risk of getting AIDS from an infected doctor, dentist or patient. There are very few cases of health professionals passing HIV to a patient. Patient-to-health-professional transmission has occurred more often. Measures are being proposed and required by medical and dental associations to decrease these possible risks, even though they are extremely low. AIDS, however, cannot be contracted by donating blood. Blood-screening tests are also done on donated blood that makes it extremely unlikely that AIDS will be transmitted in blood transfusions today. You cannot get AIDS through casual contact such as:

• Touching, holding hands or hugging
• A cough, sneeze, tears or sweat
• An animal or insect bite
• A toilet seat
• A swimming pool

Screening tests for AIDS are available from your GP or at a hospital Out-patients Department. A small sample of your blood is tested for antibodies to the HIV virus. If these antibodies are present, you test positive for and are considered infected with HIV. It could take as long as six months from exposure to the virus for these antibodies to develop. The most common reason for a false-negative test is when a person gets tested before HIV antibodies have formed. If you test positive for HIV, a second type of blood test is done to confirm it. HIV/AIDS symptoms may not develop for as long as eight to 11 years after a person is infected with the virus.

Signs and Symptoms

Early symptoms of AIDS include:
- Fatigue
- Loss of appetite
- Chronic diarrhoea
- Weight loss
- Persistent dry cough
- White spots in the mouth
- Fever
- Night sweats
- Swollen lymph glands

Persons with full-blown AIDS fall prey to many diseases such as skin infections, fungal infections, tuberculosis, pneumonia and cancer. 'Opportunistic' infections and cancer are what lead to death in an AIDS victim, not the AIDS virus itself. When the virus invades the brain cells, it leads to forgetfulness, impaired speech, trembling and seizures.

Prevention, Treatment and Care

In the future a cure for AIDS may be found. For now, prevention is the only protection. Take these steps to help avoid contracting the AIDS virus:
- Unless you are in a long-term, monogamous relationship, during sexual intercourse use condoms treated with, or along with, a spermicide containing Nonoxynol–9. (Studies suggest this spermicide may inactivate the AIDS virus.)
- Don't have sex with people who are at high risk of contracting AIDS. These have been noted to be:
  - Homosexual or bisexual men especially with multiple sex partners or who use illegal intravenous drugs
  - Heterosexual partners of persons infected or exposed to HIV
- Don't have sex with more than one person.
- Ask specific questions about your partner's sexual past, i.e., has he or she had many partners or unprotected (no-condom) sex?
- Do not be afraid to ask if he or she has been tested for HIV and if the results were positive or negative.
- Don't have sex with anyone who you know or suspect has had multiple partners. (If you've had sex with someone you suspect is HIV-positive, see your doctor.)
- Don't share needles and/or related items with anyone. This includes injecting not only illegal drugs such as heroin but also steroids, insulin, etc.

Don't have sex with people who use or have used intravenous drugs.
• Don't share personal items that have blood on them (e.g., razors).

Current treatment for AIDS includes:
• Treatment with drugs, such as AZT, which slow the virus, but do not destroy it. Hence, they may delay the onset and slow the progress of AIDS, but may have only short-term effects.
• Taking measures to reduce the risk of disease development such as adequate rest, proper nutrition and vitamin supplementation
• Emotional support
• Treating the 'opportunistic' infections that occur
AIDS is under intensive study and research. Better forms of treatment and a vaccine are being researched worldwide. A single vaccine to protect against AIDS is not very likely, though, because HIV quickly creates a new strain of the virus.

ALZHEIMER'S DISEASE

Alzheimer's disease is rare in people under 60 years of age, but it affects up to 30 per cent of people aged over 85. It is the cause of 75 per cent of all dementia cases in people over 65 years of age.

No one knows what causes Alzheimer's disease. Some research hints that a virus or infectious agent is the culprit. Others point to brain chemical deficits, a genetic predisposition and/or environmental toxins. Nevertheless, the end result is the death of brain cells that control the way your brain receives and processes information.

Signs and Symptoms

Alzheimer's disease has a gradual onset. The signs and symptoms may progress in stages. How quickly they occur varies from person to person. The disease may, however, eventually leave its victims totally unable to care for themselves.
Stage one:
• Forgetfulness
• Disorientation of time and place
• Increasing inability to do routine tasks
• Impairment of judgement
• Lessening of initiative
• Lack of spontaneity
• Depression and fear

Stage two:
• Increasing forgetfulness
• Increasing disorientation
• Wandering
• Restlessness and agitation, especially at night
• Repetitive actions
• Possible muscle twitching and/or fits

Stage three:
• Disorientation
• Inability to recognize either themselves or other people
• Speech impairment (may not be able to speak at all)
• Develop need to put everything into their mouths
• Develop need to touch everything in sight

- Become emaciated
- Complete loss of control of all body functions
  Note: The stages very often overlap.

Treatment and Care

If someone you care about shows signs of Alzheimer's disease, see that he or she gets medical attention to confirm (or rule out) the diagnosis. Problems that look like Alzheimer's may not be Alzheimer's. There are many diseases or other problems that can cause dementia – severe problems with memory and thinking. These include:

- Brain tumours
- Blood clots in the brain
- Severe vitamin B_{12} deficiency
- Hypothyroidism
- Depression
- Side effects of some medications
  Unlike Alzheimer's, these problems can be treated.

There is no known cure for Alzheimer's. Because no specific treatment or drug exists to slow the steady deterioration that typifies Alzheimer's, good planning or medical and social management are necessary to help both the victims and carers cope with the symptoms and maintain quality of life for as long as possible. It's especially helpful to put structure in the life of someone who's in the early stages of Alzheimer's. Some suggestions include:

- Maintain daily routines.
- Post reminders on a large and prominently displayed calendar.
- Make 'to do' lists of daily tasks for the person with Alzheimer's to complete, and ask him or her to check them off as they're completed.
- Put things in their proper places after use, to help the person with Alzheimer's find things when he or she needs them.
- Post safety reminders (like 'turn off the cooker') at appropriate places throughout the house.
- See that the person with Alzheimer's eats well-balanced meals, goes for walks with family members and otherwise continues to be as active as possible.

Most drug treatments currently being used are experimental. Sometimes drugs to treat depression, paranoia and agitation can minimize symptoms, but they will not necessarily improve memory.

In later stages, providing a safe environment is of the utmost importance. Alzheimer's victims should wear identification bracelets or necklaces so they can be identified should they be separated from their home environment. Seeking nursing home care for those who require supervision or medical management may be necessary.

Carers of Alzheimer's victims should be given support. They must deal with a number of financial, social, physical and emotional issues. Support for caregivers is available in many different forms, from self-help groups to periodic respite care for the sufferer.

ANGINA

Angina is a common term shortened for the medical term 'angina pectoris'. The word angina itself means pain; pectoris means chest. Angina is the chest pain or discomfort brought on by decreased circulation in the heart muscle itself. It causes a shortage of oxygen and other nutrients to the heart muscle.

Signs and Symptoms

- Squeezing pressure, heaviness or mild ache in the chest (usually behind the breastbone)
- Aching in a tooth accompanied by this squeezing pressure or heaviness in the chest
- Aching in the neck muscles or jaw
- Aching in one or both arms
- A bloated feeling in the upper abdomen and lower chest
- A choking sensation
- Paleness and sweating

These symptoms may not be extreme so they are often neglected. It is better to report an episode when these symptoms of angina occur than not to do so because you might feel foolish if something minor is causing them. Episodes of angina are usually associated with:

- Anger or excitement
- Emotional shock
- Physical work in which the discomfort goes away when the work is stopped
- Waking up at night with discomfort
- Arm use

In all of these situations, there is relief from the distress when the activity is stopped.

Many people who experience angina for the first time fear they're having a heart attack. But there are key differences between angina and a heart attack:

- A heart attack results in a damaged or injured heart muscle, angina does not. Rather, anginal pain is a warning sign of a potential heart attack. The pain indicates that the heart muscle isn't getting enough blood.
- Rest, or taking glycerol trinitrate, relieves angina, but not a heart attack.

Angina can be classified as unstable or stable:

- In unstable angina, the pain occurs without any provocation. This implies an impending heart attack and needs prompt treatment.
- In stable angina, the pain is provoked by activity and is always relieved by rest. This still needs treatment, but less urgently than unstable angina.

Contributing factors such as high blood pressure, obesity, diabetes, high cholesterol, smoking or a family history of atherosclerotic heart disease increase the chance of developing atherosclerosis and subsequent angina.

Treatment and Care

Seek emergency care for any chest pain that might be angina. Contact your doctor who will arrange appropriate investigation and treatment. The keystones of treatment are:

- Take any prescribed medicines regularly as directed. These may include drugs to lower blood pressure or to dilate (widen) the blood vessels in the heart. If you have been given a glycerol trinitrate preparation, such as tablets to put under the tongue or a spray to relieve symptoms, always carry it with you and make sure it is still within its expiry date.
- Engage in exercises to increase endurance, as advised by your doctor. (Exercise must be maintained at a level that does not cause discomfort. It may not be appropriate at all for some people.)
- Don't smoke. Nicotine in cigarettes constricts the arteries and prevents proper blood flow.
- Avoid large, heavy meals. Instead, eat lighter meals throughout the day.
- Rest after eating, or engage in some quiet activity.
- Minimize exposure to cold, windy weather.
- Lower your cholesterol level, if high, by eating a diet low in saturated fats and/or taking lipid-lowering medication, if necessary and prescribed.
- Avoid sudden strenuous exercise or other physical stress.
- Avoid anger and frustration whenever possible.

ARTHRITIS

Arthritis robs people of their freedom of movement by breaking down the protective cartilage in the joints. By destroying cartilage, arthritis results in pain and decreased movement.

Many forms of arthritis exist. The two most common forms are osteoarthritis and rheumatoid arthritis.

Osteoarthritis (OA) is a painful degeneration of the cartilage in the weight-bearing and frequently used joints. As far as researchers can tell, this kind of arthritis is typically due to a genetic predisposition plus wear and tear on the joints. It can also follow an injury to a joint. Osteoarthritis usually affects older people and is the most common type of arthritis. Brief pain and stiffness at the beginning of the day is typical.

Rheumatoid arthritis (RA) is caused by a chronic inflammation of the fingers, wrists, ankles, elbows and/or knees, causing pain, swelling and tenderness. Morning stiffness lasting longer than an hour is very common. RA affects women more often than men, striking in their 30s and 40s.

Signs and Symptoms

Symptoms of arthritis, therefore, depend on the type of arthritis that is present. Symptoms generally include:
- Stiffness
- Swelling in one or more joints
- Deep, aching pain in a joint
- Any pain associated with movement of a joint

185

- Tenderness, warmth or redness in afflicted joints
- Fever, weight loss or fatigue that accompanies joint pain

Treatment and Care

If your doctor diagnoses arthritis, he or she may prescribe medication (usually aspirin or another nonsteroidal anti-inflammatory medication), rest, heat or cold treatment and some physiotherapy or exercise, depending on what kind of arthritis you have. The goal is to reduce pain and improve joint mobility.

Among these treatments, exercise is perhaps the most important, whether it be some form of stretching, isometrics or simple endurance exercise. Exercise seems to provide both physical relief and psychological benefits. For example, it prevents the muscles from shrinking, while inactivity encourages both loss of muscle tone and bone deterioration. Too much exercise, however, will cause more pain in those with rheumatoid arthritis.

One effective and soothing form of exercise is hydrotherapy, or movement done in warm water. It allows freedom of movement and puts less stress on the joints because nearly all of the body weight is supported by the water. Doctors highly recommend swimming, too.

But remember, hydrotherapy, or any form of exercise, should never produce pain. One message that can't be emphasized enough is 'Go easy'. If you begin to feel pain, stop and rest or apply ice packs.

The following exercise suggestions may provide relief:
- Choose exercise routines that use all affected joints.
- Keep movements gradual, slow and gentle.
- If a joint is inflamed, don't exercise it.
- Don't overdo it. Allow yourself sufficient rest.
- Concentrate on freedom of movement, especially in the water, and be patient.

CANCER

Cancer refers to a broad group of diseases in which body cells grow out of control and are or become malignant (harmful).

Cancer is the second leading cause of death in the UK (heart disease is first). It affects more than one in four people in this country at some time in their lives. The most common forms are cancer of the skin, lungs, colon and rectum, breast, prostate, urinary tract and uterus.

Exactly what causes all cancers has not yet been found. Evidence suggests, however, that cancer could result from complex interactions of viruses, a person's genetic make-up, immune status and exposure to other risk factors that may promote cancer.

These risk factors include:
- Exposure to the sun's ultraviolet rays, nuclear radiation, X-rays and radon
- Use of tobacco and/or alcohol (for some cancers)
- Polluted air and water
- Dietary factors such as a high fat diet, and possibly specific food preservatives

(e.g., nitrates and nitrites) and grilled or
barbecued meats
- Exposure to a variety of chemicals
such as asbestos, benzenes, VC (vinyl
chloride), wood dust, and some
ingredients of cigarette smoke

Signs and Symptoms

Symptoms of cancer depend on the type
of cancer, the stage that it is at and
whether or not it has spread to other
parts of the body (metastasized). The
following signs and symptoms should
always be brought to your doctor's
attention because they could be warning
signals of cancer:
- Any change in bladder or bowel habits
- A lump or thickening in the breast,
testicles or anywhere else
- Unusual vaginal bleeding or rectal
discharge or any unusual bleeding
- Persistent hoarseness or nagging cough
- A sore throat that won't go away
- Noticeable change in a wart or mole
- Indigestion or difficulty swallowing

Treatment and Care

Cancer is not necessarily fatal and is, in
many cases, curable. Early detection and
proper treatment increase your chances
of surviving cancer. Early detection is
more likely if you:
- Know the warning signs of cancer and
report any of these warning signs to
your doctor if they occur.

- Do regular self-examination such as a
breast self-examination if you are a
woman (see page 137), and a testicular
self-examination if you are a man (see
page 163).
- Look at yourself in the mirror for any
noticeable changes in warts or moles or
for any wounds that have not healed.
- Take advantage of the screening
programmes which are offered to you,
such as cervical smears or mammography.
There are other screening tests available
for people who are considered to be at
high risk of developing specific tumours
(e.g., if other family members had them
or if you work or have worked in certain
jobs). Ask your doctor about this.

If and when cancer is diagnosed,
treatment will depend on the type of
cancer present, the stage it is at, and your
body's response to treatment. Cancer
treatment generally includes one or more
of the following:
- Surgery to remove the cancerous
tumour(s) and clear any obstruction to
vital passageways caused by the cancer
- Radiotherapy
- Chemotherapy
- Possibly immunotherapy

Prevention

Moreover, measures can be taken to
lower the risk of developing certain
forms of cancer:

Dietary:
- Reduce the intake of total dietary fat to
no more than 30 per cent of total

calories and reduce the intake of saturated fat to less than 10 per cent of total calories
- Eat more fruit, vegetables, and whole grains, especially:
  - Broccoli, cabbage and other vegetables in the cabbage family, including brussels sprouts. These contain cancer-fighting chemicals such as sulphoraphane and antioxidants.
  - Deep yellow-orange fruits and vegetables such as cantaloupe melons, peaches, tomatoes, carrots, sweet potatoes and very dark green vegetables such as spinach, greens and broccoli for their beta-carotene content
  - Strawberries, citrus fruits, broccoli and green peppers for vitamin C
  - Wholemeal bread, cereals, fresh fruit and vegetables and pulses for their dietary fibre content
- Strictly limit consumption of salt-cured, salt-pickled and smoked foods.
- Drink alcohol only in moderation.

Lifestyle:
- Do not smoke, use tobacco products or inhale other people's smoke.
- Limit your exposure to known carcinogens such as asbestos, radon and other workplace chemicals, as well as pesticides and herbicides.
- Have X-rays only when necessary.
- Limit your exposure to the sun's ultraviolet (UV) rays, sunlamps and tanning booths. Protect your skin from the sun's UV rays with protective clothing (e.g., sun hats and long-sleeved shirts) and sunscreen. Be sure your

sunscreen is applied frequently and contains a sun protection factor (SPF) of 15 or higher.
- Reduce stress. Emotional stress weakens the immune system, inhibiting its ability to fight off stray cancer cells.

CATARACTS

A cataract is a cloudy area in the lens or lens capsule of the eye. A cataract blocks or distorts light entering the eye. This causes problems with glare from lamps or the sun, and vision gradually becomes dull and fuzzy, even in daylight. Usually, cataracts occur in both eyes, but only one eye may be affected. If they form in both eyes, one eye can be worse than the other, because each cataract develops at a different rate. During the time cataracts are forming, vision may be helped with frequent changes in eyeglass prescriptions.

Although there are several causes of cataracts, senile cataracts are the most common form. Cataracts can accompany ageing, probably due to changes in the chemical state of lens proteins. Most people over age 65 has some degree of cataract, and almost everyone over 75 has minor visual deterioration due to cataract.

Traumatic cataracts develop after a foreign body enters the lens capsule with enough force to cause specific damage.

Complicated cataracts occur secondary to other diseases (e.g., diabetes mellitus and hypothyroidism) or other eye disorders (e.g., detached retinas, glaucoma and retinitis pigmentosa). Ionizing radiation or infra-red rays can also lead to this type of cataract.

Toxic cataracts can result from medicine or chemical toxicity. Smokers have an increased risk of developing cataracts.

Signs and Symptoms

- Cloudy, fuzzy, foggy vision
- Sensitivity to light and poor night-time vision. This can cause problems when driving at night because headlights seem too bright
- Double vision
- Pupils which are normally black appear milky white
- Seeing halos around lights
- Changes in the way you see colours
- Problems with glare from lamps or the sun
- Better vision for a while, only in long-sighted people

Prevention

- Limit exposing your eyes to X-rays, microwaves and infra-red radiation.
- Use sunglasses that block ultraviolet (UV) light.
- Wear a wide-brimmed hat or baseball cap to keep direct sunlight from your eyes while outdoors.
- Avoid overexposure to sunlight.
- Wear glasses or goggles that protect your eyes whenever you use strong chemicals, power tools or other instruments that could result in eye injury.

- Don't smoke.
- Avoid heavy drinking.
- Follow your doctor's advice to keep other illnesses such as diabetes and hypothyroidism under control.

Treatment and Care

If the vision loss caused by a cataract is only slight, surgery may not be needed. A change in your glasses, stronger bifocals or the use of magnifying lenses, and taking measures to reduce glare may help improve your vision and be sufficient for treatment. To reduce glare, wear sunglasses that filter UV light when you are out of doors. When indoors, make sure your lighting is not too bright or pointed directly at you. Use soft, white light bulbs instead of clear ones, for example, and arrange to have light reflect off walls and ceilings. When cataracts interfere with your life, however, surgery should be considered.

Modern cataract surgery is safe and effective in restoring vision. Ninety-five per cent of operations are successful. For the most part, surgery can be done as a day case or involve no more than an overnight hospital stay.

A person who has cataract surgery is usually given an artificial lens at the same time. A plastic disc called an intra-ocular lens is placed in the lens capsule inside the eye. Other choices are contact lenses and cataract glasses. Your doctor will help you to decide which choice is best for you.

It takes a couple of months for an eye to heal after cataract surgery. Experts say it is best to wait until your first eye heals before you have surgery on the second eye if it, too, has a cataract.

Following surgery, continue to protect your eyes from ultraviolet light by wearing sunglasses to filter UV rays.

CHRONIC FATIGUE SYNDROME

Other names for chronic fatigue syndrome are post-viral fatigue syndrome and myalgic encephalomyelitis (ME). It is also sometimes called 'yuppie flu' because its victims are often well-educated professionals in their 20, 30s and 40s. Many are women. Until about 1983, doctors knew next to nothing about this malady, and even today its exact cause is unknown. Early on, some researchers believed it was caused by the Epstein-Barr virus, whereas others suggested its cause could be a virus that has not yet been identified. Most experts now lean towards a theory of multiple causes.

Signs and Symptoms

Symptoms of chronic fatigue syndrome include:
- Fatigue for at least six months
- Sore throat
- Swollen lymph nodes (glands)
- Mild fever
- Headaches
- Depression
- Muscle aches
- Mild weight loss
- Short-term memory problems
- Sleep disturbances (insomnia or sleeping too much)
- Confusion, difficulty thinking, inability to concentrate

Unfortunately, these symptoms could signal any one of many diseases, and chronic fatigue syndrome can be diagnosed, therefore, only after other illnesses, such as AIDS, tuberculosis, chronic inflammatory diseases, autoimmune diseases (e.g., lupus) or psychiatric illnesses have been ruled out. There are no specific laboratory tests as yet that can diagnose the syndrome. For some, the symptoms are so debilitating that a normal working life is impossible. Yet others experience only a vague sense of feeling ill. In some cases, symptoms never let up, while in others they come and go.

Treatment and Care

Until more is known, people with chronic fatigue syndrome are encouraged to do the following:
- Get plenty of rest.
- Learn to manage stress.
- Take good care of their general health.
- Try to lead as normal a life as possible.
- Join a support group for people with this problem.

Medicines, such as paracetemol, aspirin, ibuprofen and prescribed nonsteroid anti-inflammatory drugs, may be taken to control fever and to relieve pain and muscle aches. Antidepressant drugs may also be prescribed. A gradual exercise programme, if tolerated, may also be beneficial.

CIRRHOSIS

Cirrhosis is a chronic disease of the liver. It can be caused by any injury, infection or inflammation of the liver. In cirrhosis, normal healthy liver cells are replaced with scar tissue. This prevents the liver from performing its many functions.

The liver is probably the body's most versatile organ. Among its many tasks are the following:
- Makes bile (a substance that aids in the digestion of fats)
- Produces blood proteins
- Makes chemicals which help the blood to clot
- Metabolizes cholesterol
- Helps maintain normal blood sugar levels
- Forms and stores glycogen (the body's short-term energy source)
- Manufactures more than 1,000 enzymes necessary for various bodily functions
- Detoxifies substances (e.g., alcohol and certain drugs)

The liver is equipped to handle a certain amount of alcohol without much difficulty. But too much alcohol, too often for too long causes the vital tissues in the liver to break down. Fatty deposits accumulate and scarring occurs. Cirrhosis is most commonly found in men over 45, yet the number of women developing cirrhosis is steadily increasing.

To make matters worse, people who regularly over-indulge in alcohol generally have poor nutritional habits. When alcohol replaces food, essential vitamins and minerals can be missing from the diet. Malnutrition aggravates cirrhosis.

While alcohol abuse is the most common cause of cirrhosis, hepatitis, taking certain drugs, or exposure to certain chemicals can also produce this condition.

Signs and Symptoms

Early signs and symptoms are vague but generally include:
- Poor appetite
- Nausea
- Indigestion
- Vomiting
- Weight loss
- Constipation
- Dull abdominal ache
- Fatigue

Doctors recognize the following as signs of advanced cirrhosis:
- Enlarged liver
- Yellowish eyes and skin, and dark urine (indicating jaundice)
- Bleeding from the gastro-intestinal tract
- Itching
- Hair loss
- Swelling in the legs and stomach
- Tendency to bruise easily
- Mental confusion
- Coma

Treatment and Care

Cirrhosis can be life-threatening, so get medical attention if you have any of the above symptoms. And needless to say, you (or anyone you suspect of having cirrhosis) should abstain from alcohol and get treatment for alcoholism. If you suspect some toxic substance (e.g., medicines and industrial poisons) has caused the cirrhosis, discuss the possibility with your doctor so that you can identify and eliminate the culprit.

CORONARY HEART DISEASE

The coronary arteries supply blood to the heart muscle. When they become narrow or blocked (usually by fatty deposits and/or blood clots), the heart muscle can be damaged. This is coronary heart disease (also known as coronary artery disease). Two types of coronary heart disease are angina pectoris (see angina on page 184), and acute myocardial infarction (heart attack). Myocardial infarction is the single most common cause of death in developed countries. Medical advances and growing public awareness of the benefits of exercise and good nutrition have reduced the incidence of heart disease, but there is still a long way to go. Each year in the UK, at least 250,000 people have a myocardial infarction and about 160,000 die from this cause.

Prevention

Prevention of coronary heart disease is of the utmost importance. The following steps are recommended:
• Have your blood pressure checked regularly. High blood pressure can increase the risk of atherosclerosis. To control high blood pressure, follow your doctor's advice.
• If you smoke, quit. Nicotine constricts blood flow to the heart, decreases oxygen supply to the heart and seems to play a significant role in the development of coronary heart disease.
• Be aware of the signs and symptoms of diabetes (see page 193), which is associated with atherosclerosis. Follow his or her advice if you have diabetes.
• Maintain a normal body weight. (People who are obese are more prone to atherosclerosis, high blood pressure and diabetes, and therefore coronary heart disease.)
• Eat a diet low in saturated fats and cholesterol. (Saturated fats are found in meats, dairy products with fat, hydrogenated vegetable oils and some tropical oils, like coconut and palm kernel oils). Diets high in saturated fat and cholesterol contribute to the fatty sludge that accumulates inside artery walls.
• Reduce your intake of salt.
• Take some form of exercise, such as walking, that is just sufficient to make you breathless for half an hour each day. Sitting around hour after hour, day after day, week in and week out with no regular physical activity may cause circulation problems later in life and

contributes to atherosclerosis. Start any new exercise programme gradually. Report symptoms of chest pain and/or shortness of breath to your doctor.

- Reduce the harmful effects of stress by practising relaxation techniques and improving your outlook on daily events. Stress has been linked to raised blood pressure, among other health problems.
- Get regular medical check-ups.
- Know the signs and symptoms of a heart attack so you can get immediate medical attention if necessary, before it's too late.

The signs of heart attack are:

- Chest discomfort or pressure lasting several minutes or longer
- Discomfort or pressure that spreads to the shoulder, neck, arm and jaw
- Nausea or vomiting associated with chest pain
- A cold sweat
- Difficulty breathing
- Faintness or dizziness.
- Stomach upset
- A sense of impending disaster

Treatment and Care

If you think you're having a heart attack, call your doctor or an ambulance immediately. You may need a clot-dissolving injection. If given promptly, these injections can reduce the damage to the heart. Other emergency procedures can also prevent damage to the heart.

The type of care following a heart attack will depend on the amount of damage done to the heart muscle. This can be assessed by specific medical tests and procedures. Your doctor will determine the course of treatment, which could include any or many of the following:

- Medication (cardiac, blood pressure, cholesterol-lowering drugs, etc.)
- Hospitalization for treatment and recovery from the heart attack
- Cardiac rehabilitation for lifestyle changes including: stopping smoking; losing weight; adopting a low-fat, cholesterol-controlling diet; behaviour modification; stress management; relaxation techniques
- Surgery, if appropriate: angioplasty, coronary artery bypass, etc.
- Long-term maintenance and medical follow-up

DIABETES

Diabetes is a condition that results when a person's body doesn't make any insulin or enough insulin, or is resistant to the effects of insulin. Insulin is a hormone made in the pancreas that helps your cells use blood sugar for energy. When insulin is in short supply, the glucose (sugar) in the blood can become dangerously high. That's why a person with diabetes may have to take insulin, by injection, or tablets to help the body secrete more of its own insulin or make better use of the insulin it does secrete.

Some people diagnosed as having diabetes, however, require no medication. All persons with diabetes must follow a controlled diet and exercise regularly to prevent their blood sugar from getting too high.

There are two forms of diabetes:

Type 1 – Sometimes called insulin-dependent diabetes mellitus (IDDM) or juvenile diabetes. It is the more severe type and usually develops before the age of 30 (but may occur at any age). Insulin injections, as well as dietary control and exercise, are essential.

Type 2 – Sometimes called non-insulin-dependent diabetes mellitus (NIDDM) or adult-onset diabetes. It is less severe, usually affecting persons 40 years of age or older who are overweight. This type is most often treated with diet and exercise and sometimes tablets. Occasional insulin injections may be required as well.

Diabetes can contribute to and accelerate hardening of the arteries, strokes, kidney failure and blindness.

Signs and Symptoms

The American Diabetes Association uses the acronyms DIABETES and CAUTION to help identify the warning signs of diabetes:

- **D**rowsiness
- **I**tching
- **A** family history of diabetes
- **B**lurred vision
- **E**xcessive weight
- **T**ingling, numbness or pain in extremities
- **E**asy fatigue
- **S**kin infection, slow healing of cuts and scratches, especially on the feet

Other signs are:
- **C**onstant urination
- **A**bnormal thirst
- **U**nusual hunger
- **T**he rapid loss of weight
- **I**rritability
- **O**bvious weakness and fatigue
- **N**ausea and vomiting

You don't necessarily have to experience all of these warning signs to be diabetic; only one or two may be present. Some people show no warning signs whatsoever and find out they're diabetic only after a routine blood or urine test. If you have a family history of diabetes, you should be especially watchful for the signs and symptoms listed above. If you notice any of these signs, report them to your doctor. Being overweight significantly increases your risk. A diet high in sugar and low in fibre may increase your risk as well. Pregnancy can trigger diabetes in some women.

Treatment and Care

Treatment for diabetes will depend on the type and severity of the disorder. Both forms, however, require a treatment plan that maintains normal, steady blood sugar levels. This can be accomplished by:
- Regulating the diet, with prescribed amounts of protein, fat and carbohydrates taken in regular meals, keeping these meals, and promoting weight reduction (if necessary)
- Exercise

• Medicine, in the form of oral hypoglycaemic drugs or insulin injections (if necessary)

With either type of diabetes, routine care and follow-up treatment are important. Careful control of blood sugar levels can allow a person with diabetes to lead a normal, productive life. People who are genetically predisposed to type 2 diabetes should watch their weight, control their eating habits and exercise regularly to reduce their risk of getting the disease.

DIVERTICULOSIS

No one is sure why, but sometimes small sac-like pockets protrude from the wall of the colon. This is called diverticulosis. Increased pressure within the intestines seems to be responsible. The pockets (called diverticuli) can fill with intestinal waste.

Sometimes, though, the intestinal pouches become inflamed, in which case the condition is called diverticulitis.

Many older people have diverticulosis. The digestive system becomes sluggish as a person ages. Things that increase the risk for diverticulosis include:

• Not eating enough dietary fibre. Diverticulosis is common in nations where fibre intake is low.
• Continual use of medicines that slow bowel action (e.g., painkillers, antidepressants)
• Over-use of laxatives
• Having family members who have diverticulosis

• Having gall bladder disease
• Being obese

Signs and Symptoms

In most cases, diverticulosis causes no discomfort. When there are symptoms they are usually:
• Tenderness, mild cramping or a bloated feeling usually on the lower left side of the abdomen
• Sometimes constipation or diarrhoea
• Occasionally, bright-red blood in the stools

With diverticulitis you can experience severe abdominal pain, feel nauseated and have a fever. The pain is made worse by opening the bowels. If these things occur, you should see your doctor.

Treatment and Care

Diverticular disease can't be cured, but you can reduce the discomfort and prevent complications. Eat a diet high in fibre throughout life. You can add more fibre to your diet with fresh fruit and vegetables and whole-grain foods. These pass through the system quickly, decreasing pressure in the intestines. Do, however, avoid corn, seeds and foods with seeds (e.g., figs). These are easily trapped in the troublesome pouches.

You should also drink about 1 1/2 to 2 litres (2 1/2 to 3 1/2 pints) of water every day. Avoid the regular use of stimulant laxatives (e.g., senna compounds) that make your bowel muscles contract. In fact, you should consult your doctor before taking any laxatives. If you are not able to eat a high-fibre diet, ask your doctor about taking bulk-producing laxatives like Fybogel. These are not habit-forming. Try, too, not to strain when you open your bowels. Finally, get regular exercise.

EMPHYSEMA

Can you imagine what it would feel like to breathe with a plastic bag over your head? That's exactly what emphysema feels like. This chronic lung condition greatly restricts the lives of those who suffer from it. The air sacs (alveoli) in the lungs are destroyed, and the lung loses its elasticity, along with its ability to take in oxygen. Genetic factors are responsible for 3 to 5 per cent of all cases of emphysema. Occupational and environmental exposure to irritants can also cause the disease, but the vast majority of people with emphysema are cigarette smokers aged 50 or older. In fact, emphysema is sometimes called the smoker's disease because of its strong link with cigarettes.

Signs and Symptoms

Emphysema takes a number of years to develop, and early symptoms can be easily missed. Symptoms to look out for include:
• Shortness of breath on exertion
• Wheezing
• Fatigue

• Slight body build with marked weight loss and barrel chest
• Breathing through pursed lips
(Note: Persons with emphysema experiencing severe symptoms may need emergency care.)

Emphysema is often accompanied by chronic bronchitis. Persons with chronic bronchitis have symptoms of coughing and production of excess sputum.

Treatment and Care

A doctor can diagnose emphysema based on your medical history, a physical examination, a chest X-ray, and a lung-function test (spirometry). By the time emphysema is detected, however, anywhere from 50 to 70 per cent of the lung tissue may already be destroyed. At this point, your doctor may recommend the following:
• A programme for stopping smoking
• Avoidance of other people's smoke (passive smoking)
• Avoidance of dust, fumes, pollutants and other irritating inhalants
• Physiotherapy to help loosen mucus in your lungs (if chronic bronchitis accompanies the emphysema)
• Daily exercise
• A diet that includes adequate amounts of all essential nutrients
• Prescription medication which may include a bronchodilator, steroids and antibiotics
• Annual flu vaccinations
• A supply of oxygen at home either from cylinders or from an oxygen concentrator

Emphysema is irreversible, however, so prevention is the only real way to avoid permanent damage.

EPILEPSY

Epilepsy is a disorder of the brain. For some reason, with epilepsy there is excessive electrical activity in nerve cells in the brain. Some of the known causes of epilepsy include:
- Brain damage, either at birth or from a severe head injury
- Alcohol or drug abuse
- Brain infection
- Brain tumour

More often than not, however, the cause is not known. Epilepsy affects people of all ages, male and female. It often begins in childhood or adolescence, and while the disorder tends to run in families, epilepsy is not contagious.

Signs and Symptoms

The most common symptom is a seizure, of which there are several types. The type depends on the part of the brain the seizure starts in, how fast it takes place and how wide an area of the brain it involves.
- Grand mal or tonic-clonic seizures. There can be many symptoms, including crying out, falling down, losing consciousness, entire body stiffening, then uncontrollable jerks and twitches. The sufferer's muscles relax after the seizure. He or she may lose bowel and bladder control and may be be confused, sleepy and have a headache after the seizure.
- Petit mal or absence seizures. Symptoms include staring into space and repeated blinking. The sufferer is unaware of the seizure, but someone else may think he or she is daydreaming or not paying attention. These seizures can occur once a day, or more than a hundred times a day. They occur most often in children and can result in learning problems.
- Partial seizures. These are less common than grand mal or petit mal seizures. They include:
  - Simple ones, of which the symptoms include tingling feelings, twitching, seeing flashing lights, hallucination of smell and/or taste
  - Complex ones, which involve episodes (e.g., sitting motionless or moving or behaving in strange or repetitive ways) called automatisms. Examples include lip smacking, chewing, and fidgeting with the hands. There is usually no loss of consciousness, but the person who has this type of seizure may be confused and not remember details of it.

Treatment and Care

A medical diagnosis is necessary and will include:
- Information about the attacks. This may need to be given by someone else because the sufferer is often not aware of what has happened.

197

• A complete neurological exam which includes a test to measure the electrical activity of the brain (EEG). Specialized imaging tests (e.g., computerized tomography [CT] scans and magnetic resonance imaging [MRI] scans) and blood tests may also be done.

Persons with recurrent seizures are usually given anticonvulsant drugs to prevent or lessen the chance of future seizures. Epileptics can lead normal lives once the seizures are controlled by medicine or do not occur for several years. This, however, depends on the type of seizure. Persons with general convulsive seizures may have restrictions placed on driving and high-risk activities (e.g., certain jobs, sports, anything involving heights, using dangerous machinery or being in any potentially hazardous situation). If medication is not effective and the seizures are confined to a specific single area of the brain, in rare cases, surgery may be performed.

GALLSTONES

Gallstones are stone deposits of a mixture of cholesterol (the same fat-like substance that clogs arteries), bilirubin and protein that are found in the gallbladder or bile ducts. These stones can range in size from less than a pinhead to 7–8 cm (about 3 in) across. Gallstones are up to four times as common in women as in men and become more common with age. It is estimated that 20 per cent of all women develop gallstones.

Depending on their size and location, gallstones may cause no symptoms or may require medical treatment.

Doctors aren't sure why gallstones form, but some people are clearly more susceptible than others. Factors that encourage gallstones to form include:
• A family history of gallbladder disease
• Obesity
• Middle age
• Being female
• Pregnancy
• Taking oestrogen
• Diabetes
• Eating a diet high in cholesterol-rich foods
• Diseases of the small intestine

Signs and Symptoms

Symptoms of gallstones include:
• Feeling bloated and having wind, especially after eating fried or fatty foods
• Steady pain in the upper right abdomen that lasts from 20 minutes to five hours
• Pain between the shoulder blades or in the right shoulder
• Indigestion, nausea, vomiting
• Severe abdominal pain with fever and sometimes yellow skin and/or eyes (jaundice)

Treatment and Care

Treatments for gallstones range from:
• Dietary measures (e.g., a low-fat diet) to reduce contractions of the gallbladder, thus limiting pain

- Medications to dissolve the stones
- Lithotripsy (the use of shock waves to shatter the stones)
- Surgery to remove the gallbladder

GLAUCOMA

Glaucoma happens when the pressure of the liquid in the eye gets too high and causes damage. Glaucoma tends to run in families and is one of the most common major eye disorders in people over the age of 60. In fact, the risk of getting glaucoma increases with age, but it can also be triggered or aggravated by some medicines like antihistamines and antispasmodics.

Signs and Symptoms

There are two types of glaucoma:
- Chronic or open-angle glaucoma. This type develops gradually and in the early stages usually causes no pain and no symptoms. When signs and symptoms begin, they include:
  - Loss of side (peripheral) vision
  - Blurred vision
  In the late stages, symptoms include:
  - Vision loss in larger areas (side and central vision) usually in both eyes
  - Blind spots
  - Seeing halos around lights
  - Poor night vision
  - Blindness if not treated early enough
- Acute or angle-closure glaucoma. This type can occur suddenly and is a medical emergency!

Signs and symptoms include:
- Severe pain in and above the eye
- Severe throbbing headache
- Fogginess of vision, halos around lights
- Redness in the eye, swollen upper eyelid
- Dilated pupil
- Nausea, vomiting, weakness

Treatment and Care

Glaucoma may not be preventable, but the blindness that may result from it is. Ask to be tested for glaucoma whenever you have a routine eye test. It's a simple, painless procedure. If pressure inside the eyeball is high, an eye specialist (ophthalmologist) will probably give you eye drops and perhaps oral medicines. The aim of both is to reduce the pressure inside the eye.

Medicines given for acute glaucoma are prescribed for life. If you have glaucoma, let your doctor know or remind him or her of any medicines you take.

Also, do not take any medicine – even nonprescription ones – without first checking with your doctor or pharmacist. Most cold medications and sleeping pills, for example, can cause the pupil in the eye to dilate. This can lead to increased eye pressure, which can worsen glaucoma.

If medicines do not control the pressure, laser beam surgery and other surgical procedures are available. These widen the drainage channels within the eye and relieve fluid build-up.

There are also some things you can do for yourself:

- Avoid getting upset and fatigued. They can increase pressure in the eye.
- Don't smoke cigarettes. It causes blood vessels to constrict which reduces blood supply to the eye.

GOUT

Gout is a form of arthritis most common in men older than 30 and in women after the menopause and is caused by increased blood levels of uric acid, produced by the breakdown of protein in the body. When blood levels of uric acid rise above a critical level, thousands of hard, tiny uric acid crystals collect in the joints. These crystals act like tiny, hot, jagged shards of glass, resulting in pain and inflammation. Crystals can collect in the tendons and cartilage, in the kidneys (as kidney stones) and in the fatty tissues beneath the skin. Gout can strike any joint, but often affects those in the feet such as the big toe, and those in the legs.

A gout attack can last several hours to a few days. People who have gout can be symptom-free for years between attacks. Gout can be triggered by:

- Mild trauma or blow to the joint
- Drinking alcohol (beer and wine more so than spirits)
- Eating a diet rich in red meat (especially offal such as liver, kidney or tongue)
- Eating sardines or anchovies
- Taking certain drugs (e.g., diuretics)

Signs and Symptoms

- Excruciating pain and inflammation in a joint or joints that strikes suddenly and peaks quickly
- Affected area which is swollen, red, feels warm, and is very tender to the touch
- Feeling of agonizing pain after even the slightest pressure such as a sheet rubbing against the affected area
- Sometimes a mild fever and chills

Treatment and Care

Never assume you have gout without consulting a doctor. Many conditions can mimic an acute attack of gout, including infection, injury or rheumatoid arthritis. Only a doctor can accurately diagnose your problem.

If you do have gout, treatment will depend on the reasons for your high levels of uric acid. Your doctor can conduct a simple test to determine if your kidneys aren't clearing uric acid from the blood the way they should or to determine whether your body simply produces too much uric acid.

The first goal is to relieve the acute gout attack. The second goal is to prevent a recurrence.

- For immediate relief, your doctor will prescribe a nonsteroidal anti-inflammatory medication or other painkiller and tell you to rest the affected joint.
- For long-term relief, your doctor will probably recommend that you lose

excess weight, limit your intake of alcohol, drink plenty of liquids and take medication, if necessary. The commonest type of medication is allopurinol, which decreases uric acid production. Another (probenecid) increases the excretion of uric acid from the kidneys.

HIGH BLOOD PRESSURE

High blood pressure (hypertension) isn't like toothache, a bruise or constipation. Nothing hurts, looks discolored or fails to work. Usually, people with high blood pressure experience no discomfort or outward signs of trouble. Yet high blood pressure is a silent killer. Uncontrolled high blood pressure increases the risk of heart attack, stroke, kidney failure or loss of vision.

High blood pressure occurs when your blood moves through your arteries at a higher pressure than normal. The heart is actually straining to pump blood through the arteries. This isn't healthy because:

• It promotes hardening of the arteries (atherosclerosis). Hardened, narrowed arteries may not be able to carry the amount of blood the body's organs need.

• Blood clots can form or lodge in a narrowed artery. (This could cause a stroke or heart attack.)

• The heart can become enlarged and might subsequently fail, as occurs in congestive heart failure.

More than half of all older adults have high blood pressure. About 50 per cent of all people who have it don't know it. Worse yet, many people who know their blood pressure is dangerously high are doing nothing to try to control it. And for 90 per cent of those affected, there is no known cause. When this is the case, it is called primary or essential hypertension. When high blood pressure results from another medical disorder or a drug it is referred to as secondary hypertension. In these cases (about 10 per cent of total), the blood pressure goes back to normal if the root cause is corrected.

Detection

How's your blood pressure? Blood pressure is normally measured with a blood-pressure cuff (sphygmomanometer) placed on the arm. The numbers on the gauge measure your blood pressure in millimetres of mercury (mmHg). The first (higher) number measures the systolic pressure. This is the maximum pressure exerted against the arterial walls during a heart beat. The second (lower) number records the diastolic pressure, the pressure between heart beats, when the heart is resting. The results are then recorded as systolic/diastolic pressure (120/80 mmHg, for example). Blood pressure is considered high in adults if it is consistently a reading of 140 mmHg systolic and/or 90 mmHg diastolic or higher.

To determine your blood pressure accurately, an average of two or more readings should be taken on two or more separate occasions. If your blood pressure is generally pretty good and suddenly registers high, don't be alarmed. Anxiety and other strong emotions, physical exertion, drinking a large amount of coffee, or digesting a recently consumed meal can temporarily elevate normal blood pressure with no lasting effects. If, after several readings, your doctor is convinced you do indeed have high blood pressure, follow his or her advice.

Treatment and Care

The amazing part is, blood pressure is one of the easiest health problems to control. Here's a multi-faceted plan to control high blood pressure:
- If you're overweight, lose weight.
- Don't smoke.
- Limit alcohol to two drinks or less a day.
- Reduce your salt intake. (This is helpful for many people.)
- Use salt substitutes if your doctor recommends this.
- Take daily exercise that is sufficient to make you slightly short of breath for half an hour.
- Learn to handle stress by practising relaxation techniques and rethinking stressful situations.
- Take any prescribed blood pressure medicine as directed.
- Don't skip your pills because you feel fine or because you don't like the side effects. Tell your doctor if you have any side effects of the medicine such as dizziness, faintness, skin rash or a dry cough in the absence of a cold. Another medicine can be prescribed.

- Talk to your doctor or pharmacist before you take antihistamines and decongestants. An ingredient in some of these can raise your blood pressure.

KIDNEY STONES

Kidney stones are hard masses of mineral deposits (e.g., calcium) or other organic substances (e.g., uric acid) that form in the kidneys or urinary tract. They can be found in the kidney itself or anywhere in the ureter (the tube that carries urine from the kidney to the bladder). Kidney stones can be as small as a tiny pebble or 2–3 cm (1 in) or more in diameter. They are more common in men (especially between 30 and 50 years old) than in women or children.

Signs and Symptoms

Kidney stones can be present for many years without causing symptoms. When a stone becomes large enough to produce problems, the following symptoms may occur:
- Blocked flow of urine
- Frequent and painful urination
- Blood in the urine
- Nausea and vomiting
- Fever, chills
- Severe pain and tenderness over the affected area
- Pain that can be agonizing and radiate down the side of the abdomen and into the groin area when the stone becomes lodged in the ureter

(Note: If these symptoms are severe, emergency care may be needed.)

Treatment and Care

Treatment will depend on the size, symptoms, location and cause of the kidney stone(s). The doctor will take urine and blood samples and request ultrasound and/or X-rays to determine the location and type of stone present. If the stone is small and can be passed, treatment consists of drinking plenty of fluids.

A range of different procedures can be used to remove the stones:

• Open surgery. This has been super-seded for many cases by other options.
• Endoscopic surgery. A cystoscope (a type of endoscope for viewing the bladder) is passed, with attachments for gripping or crushing the stone, through the urethra into the bladder.
• Laparoscopic surgery. This is similar to the previous option, but the viewing instrument and attachments are passed through a small opening made in the skin of the abdomen.
• Lithotripsy. In this procedure, shock waves are used to break the stone down into small pieces which can then be passed in the urine. Not all stones are suitable for this treatment.

Kidney stones can and do recur. If you're prone to developing stones, follow these guidelines:

• Save any stones you pass so your doctor can have them analysed.

(Treatment varies with the type of stones you form.)

• Follow your doctor's dietary advice. If you tend to form calcium stones, he or she will probably advise you to limit your calcium intake. If you form uric acid stones, your doctor may recommend that you eat less protein.
• Drink plenty of fluids – preferably 2–3 litres ($3^1/_2$–$5^1/_2$ pints) of water daily and more than this in hot weather.
• See your doctor regularly to be sure your kidneys are functioning as they should.

LUNG CANCER

Lung cancer is the most common cancer in the UK. It is the most common cause of cancer deaths in men, and the second most common cause of cancer deaths in women (after breast cancer). The incidence of lung cancer in women has shown a marked increase in the last decade due to an increase in women smokers. Lung cancer currently causes a total of around 35,000 deaths each year. It is uncommon before the age of 40 and is most common between 65 and 75. Besides cigarette smoke, other factors that increase the risk of getting lung cancer are exposure to radon, asbestos or other environmental pollutants.

Lung cancer is especially deadly because the rich network of blood vessels that deliver oxygen from the lungs to the rest of the body can also spread cancer very quickly. By the time it's diagnosed, other organs may be affected.

Signs and Symptoms

Symptoms of lung cancer include:
- Chronic cough
- Blood-streaked sputum
- Shortness of breath
- Wheezing
- Chest discomfort with each breath
- Weight loss
- Fatigue

Treatment, Care and Prevention

Lung cancer is difficult to detect in its early, more treatable stages, so the best way to combat the disease is to prevent it. As you might guess, the first step is to eliminate the single greatest cause of lung cancer – smoking cigarettes.

The risk of developing lung cancer is proportional to the number of cigarettes smoked per day. Also, the longer a person smokes and the more deeply the smoke is inhaled, the greater the risk of getting lung cancer.

You should also avoid or limit exposure to environmental pollutants. If you are in a risk area, you can have your home tested for radon.

Depending on the type of lung cancer and how far it has spread, the diseased portions of the lung may be surgically removed. For some people, radiotherapy or chemotherapy (or both) will be needed instead of or in addition to surgery.

MACULAR DEGENERATION

Macular degeneration is a common cause of blindness for those over 55 years of age. The central part of the retina (the macula) deteriorates, leading to loss of central, or straight-ahead, vision. One or both eyes may be affected.

The exact cause is not known. In many cases, though, the small vessels of the eye have become narrowed and hardened due to atherosclerosis. When this happens, the macula doesn't get the blood supply it needs, which in turn causes it to degenerate, or waste away. This is called the dry form. In the wet form (which is less common than the dry), tiny blood vessels leak blood or fluid around the macula.

Signs and Symptoms

Macular degeneration is painless. It usually develops gradually, especially the dry form. With the wet form, symptoms can occur more rapidly. Symptoms for both forms are:
- Blurred or cloudy vision
- Seeing a dark or blind spot at the centre of vision
- Distorted vision such as straight lines that look wavy
- Difficulty reading or doing other close-up work
- Difficulty doing any activity that requires sharp vision (e.g., driving)
- Complete loss of central vision. Peripheral, or side, vision is not affected.

Treatment and Care

If you notice any of the signs and symptoms of macular degeneration, you should see your doctor or optician right away. Laser treatment, if performed before much damage is done to the eyesight, may help to slow the progress if you have the wet form of this condition. Most dry form cases are not treatable, but vision can be helped by special powerful glasses if they are worn in the early course of the condition.

MULTIPLE SCLEROSIS

The nervous system carries messages to and from the rest of your body. Normally, delicate nerves are encased in a protective covering called myelin. With multiple sclerosis, the myelin becomes inflamed and eventually dissolves. Over time, scar tissue (sclerosis) develops where the myelin used to be, in scattered locations in the brain and spinal cord. Nerve impulses, which normally travel at a speed of 225 miles per hour, either slow down considerably or come to a complete halt. People most susceptible to MS are:

- White adults between 20 and 40 years of age
- Those whose siblings or parents already have the disease
- Women (at a ratio of three women to every two men)
- Residents of northern Europe, the northern United States and Canada

No one knows what causes MS, but infection and other immunity factors are possibilities. Some theories point to toxins, trauma, nutritional deficiencies and other factors that lead to the destruction of myelin as possible causes. Overwork, fatigue, the period soon after giving birth for women, acute infections and fevers have been known to precede the onset of multiple sclerosis but don't cause it.

Signs and Symptoms

Early signs and symptoms may be mild and present for years before a diagnosis of multiple sclerosis is made. Once diagnosed, the symptoms may last for hours or weeks, vary from day to day, and come and go with no predictable pattern. Symptoms include:
- Fatigue
- Weakness
- Numbness
- Muscle spasticity (muscles which are stiff and difficult to control)
- Poor coordination (trembling of the hand, for example)
- Bladder problems (frequent urination, urgency, infection and incontinence)
- Blurred vision or double vision
- Transient blindness in one eye
- Emotional mood swings, irritability, depression, anxiety, euphoria

Treatment and Care

While no cure exists for multiple sclerosis, several steps can be taken to

make living with the disease easier. These include:
- Getting plenty of rest
- Treating bacterial infections and fever as soon as they occur
- Minimizing stressful situations, especially physically demanding ones, since physical stress may aggravate the symptoms
- Staying out of the heat and sun since an increased body temperature can aggravate MS symptoms
- Avoiding hot showers or baths, since they, too, can aggravate symptoms. In fact, cool baths or swimming in a pool may lessen symptoms by lowering body temperature.
- Maintaining a normal routine at work and at home if activities aren't physically demanding
- Getting regular exercise (physiotherapy may be helpful)
- Having body massages to help maintain muscle tone
- Getting professional, supportive psychological counselling
- Taking prescribed medication. This may include:
  - injections of beta interferon
  - short-term courses of cortisone-like drugs such as intravenous (IV) or oral steroids
  - antispasmodics
  - muscle relaxants
  - antidepressants
  - antianxiety drugs
  - antibiotics (to treat any bacterial infections)
  - medications to control urinary function

OSTEOPOROSIS

Osteoporosis (reduction in bone mass and strength, making the bones brittle and more prone to fracture) is a normal part of the aging process. Peak bone mass is reached between the ages of 25 and 35 years. After 35, everyone's bones lose density. By the age of 70, the skeleton is typically about one third as dense as at its peak. In some people, excessive thinning of the bones occurs and this becomes a serious medical problem. Any bone can be affected by osteoporosis, but the hips, wrists and spine are the most common sites.

The actual causes of osteoporosis are unknown. Certain risk factors, however, increase the likelihood of developing significant osteoporosis. Women are four times more likely to be affected than men.

The reasons are as follows:
- Their bones are generally thinner and lighter to start with.
- They live longer than men.
- They have rapid bone loss at the menopause due to a sharp decline of oestrogen. (The risk also increases for women who experience the menopause before age 45 naturally or as a result of surgery which removes the ovaries, and also for women who experience a lack of or irregular menstrual flow.)

Risk factors for women and men:
- Having a thin, small-framed body
- Race. Caucasians and Asians are at a higher risk than Afro-Caribbeans.

- Lack of physical activity, especially walking, running, tennis and other weight-bearing exercises.
- Lack of calcium. Adequate calcium intake throughout life helps to prevent calcium deficiency that contributes to a weakening of bone mass.
- Heredity. The risk increases if there is a history of osteoporosis and/or bone fractures in your family.
- Cigarette smoking
- Alcohol – Regularly consuming alcoholic drinks may be damaging to bones. Heavy drinkers often have poor nutrition and may be more prone to fractures due to their predisposition to falls.
- Taking certain medications such as corticosteroids (anti-inflammatory drugs used to treat a variety of conditions such as asthma, arthritis and lupus) can lead to bone-tissue loss. Some anticonvulsive drugs may also increase the risk.
- Other disorders such as overactivity of the thyroid and parathyroid glands and certain forms of bone cancer can also increase the risk.

Signs and Symptoms

Osteoporosis is a 'silent disease' because it can progress without any noticeable signs or symptoms. Often the first sign is when a bone fracture occurs. Symptoms include:
- A gradual loss of height
- A rounding of the shoulders
- Acute lower backache
- Swelling of a wrist after a fall

Treatment and Care

Medical tests such as bone densitometry can measure bone mass in various sites of the body. They are safe and painless. These tests can help doctors decide if and what kind of treatment is needed. Treatment for osteoporosis includes:
- Dietary measures: a balanced diet rich in calcium plus calcium supplements if necessary
- Daily exercises approved by your doctor
- Fall prevention strategies:
  - Use grab bars and safety mats or nonskid tape in your bath or shower.
  - Use handrails on stairs.
  - Don't stoop to pick things up. Pick things up by bending your knees and keeping your back straight.
  - Wear flat, sturdy, non-skid shoes.
  - If you use rugs, make sure they have non-skid backs.
  - Use a stick or walking frame if necessary.
  - See that halls, stairs and entrances are well-lit. Put a night-light in your bathroom.
- Proper posture
- Medical management – There are a number of medical treatments available. Women benefit from hormone replacement therapy (HRT), particularly if given at the onset of the menopause. Calcitonin or biphosphonates are also prescribed for some people.
- Surgery (such as hip replacement) if necessary

Prevention

To prevent or slow osteoporosis, take these steps now:

- Be sure to eat a balanced diet including adequate daily intakes of calcium. The recommended daily allowance (RDA) is 800 milligrams a day for most adults, and 1500 milligrams a day for postmenopausal women not on hormone replacement therapy. Typical intakes are only 500 milligrams for women and 700 milligrams for men.
- To get your recommended calcium, choose these high-calcium foods daily:
  - Milk, yogurt and cheese (low-fat options will keep your fat intake down)
  - Soft-boned fish and shellfish such as salmon, sardines, prawns
  - Vegetables, especially broccoli and kale
  - Beans and bean sprouts as well as tofu (soya bean curd, if processed with calcium)
  - Calcium-fortified foods such as some orange juices, apple juices and ready-to-eat cereals
- Check with your doctor before taking calcium supplements.
- Follow a programme of regular, weight-bearing exercise (e.g., walking, jogging, low-impact or non-impact aerobics) at least three or four times a week.
- Do not smoke. Smoking makes osteoporosis worse and may negate the beneficial effects of oestrogen replacement therapy.
- Limit alcohol consumption.
- Check with your doctor regarding medical management to prevent and treat osteoporosis especially if you are at a high risk of getting the disorder. HRT may help if you are a woman. There are risks with HRT, though, so you need to check with your doctor to see how they apply to you.

PARKINSON'S DISEASE

Parkinson's disease is a nervous system disorder. It causes tremors in which there is involuntary shaking in the limbs and head, a shuffling gait and stiffness. With it comes a gradual, progressive stiffness of muscles.

Parkinson's disease most often strikes people over 60 years of age. The exact cause of Parkinson's disease is not known, but what is known is that it results from the degeneration of cells in the part of the brain that produces dopamine, a substance which nerves need to function properly.

Signs and Symptoms

The signs and symptoms of Parkinson's disease include:

- Slow or stiff movement
- Stooped posture
- Shuffling or dragging of the feet
- Tremors and shaking of the head
- Monotonic voice, weak and high-pitched
- Blinking less frequently than normal
- Lack of spontaneity in facial expression
- Problems in swallowing
- Difficulty in adjusting positions
- Depression and anxiety
- Dementia (in advanced stages)

Treatment and Care

Parkinson's disease is not yet curable. Great strides, however, have been made in treatment, offering new hope for the 270,000 or so people affected by this condition in the UK. For the most part, symptoms can be relieved or controlled. Parkinson's disease does not significantly lower life expectancy.

Medications containing L-dopa increase the dopamine level in the brain. For many people, these medicines control symptoms. Other medicines are available to be used with L-dopa or as an alternative to it if symptoms are not controlled.

Other treatments try to make the person with Parkinson's more comfortable. Warm baths and massages, for example, can help prevent muscle rigidity. Here are some other helpful hints:

- Take care to maintain a safe home environment. For example, replace razor blades with electric shavers, use non-skid rugs and handrails to prevent falls.
- Simplify tasks. Replace laced shoes with slip-ons, for instance, or wear clothing that can be pulled on or that have zips or velcro strips instead of buttons.
- Include high-fibre foods in the diet and drink plenty of fluids to prevent constipation.
- Physiotherapy often helps.
- Remain as active as possible.
- Get professional help to relieve depression, if necessary.

PEPTIC ULCERS

Ulcers located in the stomach (gastric ulcers) and ulcers in the first section of the small intestine (duodenal ulcers), are grouped under the label peptic ulcers. They afflict men, women and children. No one knows exactly what causes ulcers, but doctors think they're a combination of excess stomach acid and failure of the stomach's inner lining to protect it from the acid. Also, bacteria called *Heliobacter pylori* are known to cause ulcers.

Tests can be performed by your doctor to find out if you have this bacteria. They include a blood test, a breath test or a biopsy of stomach tissue obtained by endoscopy. If *Heliobacter pylori* bacteria are present, antibiotics should be prescribed.

One study has shown that treating ulcers of this type protected nearly 90 per cent of those affected from future ulcer attacks. Another showed that only 15 per cent of people with ulcers that were treated with *Heliobacter pylori* had recurrent ulcers after two years. People with a family history of ulcers tend to be a greater risk for developing an ulcer as do people with type O blood. In 80 to 90 per cent of cases, peptic ulcers recur within two years of the initial attack.

Certain things increase the risk of peptic ulcers in susceptible individuals:
- Stress and anxiety
- Irregular meal times or skipping meals, and improper diet
- Excess alcohol, drugs and caffeine, which irritate the stomach

Signs and Symptoms

Peptic ulcers are characterized by:
- A gnawing or burning sensation just above the navel within $1\frac{1}{2}$ to 3 hours after eating
- Pain that frequently causes waking at night
- Pain generally relieved within minutes by food or antacids
- Pain that recurs, with each cluster of attacks lasting from several days to several months
- Pain that feels like indigestion, heartburn or hunger
- Nausea
- Unintentional weight loss or loss of appetite
- Anaemia

Treatment and Care

Doctors can diagnose gastric and duodenal ulcers on the basis of X-rays or endoscopy (looking at your stomach through a tube that's inserted via your mouth).

Notify your doctor if:
- Your stools are ever bloody, black or tarry-looking. (Take a specimen to your doctor's surgery.)
- You vomit blood or material that looks like coffee grounds
- You become unusually pale and weak
- You have diarrhoea with intolerable pain

For treatment, your doctor may prescribe:
- Over-the-counter antacids
- A combination of antibiotics and acid-suppressing agents if he or she thinks that Heliobacter pylori bacteria is contributing to your ulcer.
- Medicines to decrease or stop the stomach's production of hydrochloric acid or medicine to coat the ulcer, protecting it from the acid so it has time to heal
- Surgery to cut the nerves that stimulate acid production or to remove part of the stomach. This is rarely needed but may be tried if other treatment methods fail.

If you have an ulcer, you can soothe the pain in various ways. Some suggestions are:
- Eat smaller, lighter, more frequent meals for a couple of weeks. Big, heavy lunches and dinners can spell trouble for people with ulcers. Frequent meals tend to take the edge off pain.
- Avoid anything that will stimulate excess stomach acid. This includes coffee, tea, alcohol and soft drinks containing caffeine. Even decaffeinated coffee should be avoided because it can cause heartburn.
- Discontinue use of aspirin and other nonsteroidal anti-inflammatory medicine, which irritate the stomach lining.
- Try antacids (with your doctor's approval) on a short-term basis. Drugs which suppress acid production are now available over the counter. If your symptoms return after completing a course of these drugs, you should see your doctor.
- Don't smoke. Smokers get ulcers more frequently than non-smokers. No one is sure why.

• Try to minimize stress in your life. Stress doesn't cause ulcers. But for some people, stress triggers the release of stomach acid – and subsequent ulcer flare-ups.

PHLEBITIS

The medical term for this condition is thrombophlebitis. In it, a vein, usually in the leg, becomes inflamed due to the formation of small blood clots. The problem is usually caused by infection or injury. Phlebitis is more common in women than in men.

Signs and Symptoms

Symptoms of phlebitis depend on its type:
• Superficial phlebitis affects the veins visible just beneath the skin surface. It often affects people who have varicose veins. The affected area will be red and swollen and feel warm, hard and tender to the touch. Usually responsive to home treatment, this type seldom results in clots that break loose and flow into the bloodstream.
• Deep vein thrombophlebitis, by contrast, can result in a blood clot that breaks away from the wall of a vein. This then goes into the circulation and may lodge in the lung (pulmonary embolism). This type of phlebitis may occur after prolonged bed rest, major surgery, a heart attack or a stroke. The only symptom may be an aching pain in the limb, but 50 per cent of people with

deep vein thrombophlebitis have no symptoms. Others may have severe leg pain with swelling of the lower leg.

Other conditions that can increase the risk of phlebitis of either kind include:
• General inactivity (from a sedentary job, after a prolonged trip by car or plane, or following surgery)
• Smoking or chewing tobacco
• Being overweight
• Trauma to the leg (from a blow or fall)
• Injury to the vein (from injections or intravenous needles)
• Some malignancies
• Advancing age

Treatment and Care

Only a medical professional can tell the difference between superficial and deep vein types. If you're diagnosed as having superficial phlebitis, you'll probably be told to:
• Rest the affected limb and elevate it until the pain and swelling subside.
• Apply moist heat to the affected area for 20 minutes on and 20 minutes off.
• Take aspirin or nonsteroidal anti-inflammatory medications (e.g., ibuprofen). *Note: Do not give aspririn, or any medication containing salicylates, to children under 12 years of age, unless directed by a doctor, due to its association with Reye's syndrome, a potentially fatal condition.*
Deep vein thrombophlebitis requires hospitalization and treatment with blood-thinning drugs to prevent an embolism

from forming. If you notice any symptoms of this type, especially severe leg pain and swelling of the lower leg, see your doctor.

Prevention

- Avoid prolonged periods of uninterrupted sitting or standing.
- Avoid smoking if you take birth control pills or oestrogen medication.
- Avoid sitting with your legs crossed.
- Avoid wearing garters, knee-high hosiery or other stockings that restrict blood flow in the legs.
- Wear properly fitting elasticated stockings made to help blood flow in the legs.
- Exercise your legs at least every hour or two on long car or plane trips.
- If you're confined to bed, move your feet and ankles around for at least five minutes in every hour.

PNEUMONIA

Pneumonia is inflammation of the lungs due to infection. It is the certified cause of death for about 27,000 people a year in the UK. It is often a complication of another serious illness.

Pneumonia can develop when the lungs are infected by either bacteria, viruses, fungi or toxins, causing inflammation. Certain people are at a greater risk of developing pneumonia than others. They include:

- Elderly people, because the body's ability to fight off disease diminishes with age
- People who are hospitalized for other conditions
- Individuals with a suppressed cough reflex following a stroke
- Smokers, because tobacco smoke paralyses the tiny hairs that otherwise help to expel germ-ridden mucus from the lungs
- People who suffer from malnutrition, alcoholism or viral infections
- Anyone with a recent respiratory viral infection
- People with emphysema or chronic bronchitis
- People with sickle-cell anaemia
- Cancer patients undergoing radiotherapy or chemotherapy, both of which depress the immune system
- People with HIV (human immune deficiency virus)

Signs and Symptoms

Pneumonia symptoms include:
- Chest pain (may worsen when inhaling)
- Fever and chills
- Coughing with little or no sputum or sometimes with bloody, dark yellow or rust-colored sputum
- Difficulty in breathing, rapid breathing
- General fatigue, headache, nausea, vomiting

Treatment, Care and Prevention

Treatment for pneumonia will depend on its type (viral, bacterial or chemical, for example) and location. X-rays, sputum analysis and blood tests can help identify these. Treatment includes:

- Getting plenty of bed rest
- Using steam inhalations
- Drinking plenty of fluids
- Taking paracetamol to relieve minor discomfort and reduce fever
- Taking any medications your doctor prescribes: antibiotics to treat bacterial pneumonia or to fight a secondary bacterial infection; antiviral medicines, if indicated; nose drops, sprays or oral decongestants to treat congestion in the upper respiratory tract.
- Cough medicines as needed: a cough suppressant for a dry, unproductive cough; an expectorant type for a mucus-producing cough
- Removing fluid from the lungs by suction. Anti-inflammatory medications and oxygen therapy may be used for chemically induced pneumonias.
- Also, vaccination against influenza is recommended for people aged 65 and older and for people suffering from chronic diseases such as diabetes or heart or lung disease. Ask your doctor about them.

SCOLIOSIS

Scoliosis generally appears between the ages of 10 and 15, and affects girls seven to nine times more often than boys. In most cases, no one knows the cause.

In the beginning, scoliosis isn't painful. But it slowly twists the upper portion of the spine. One shoulder may curve one way while the lower back twists another, so that the chest and back are distorted. The spine begins to rotate, and one side of the rib cage becomes more prominent. This is more obvious if the person bends forwards at the waist, with the arms hanging freely. A doctor will be able to detect scoliosis by asking a patient to assume such a position during a routine physical examination or screening for scoliosis.

Signs and Symptoms

Any of the following may indicate scoliosis:

- An uneven hemline or unequal trouser legs
- One hip higher than the other
- One shoulder higher than the other or one shoulder blade sticks out (noticeable when the shirt is off)
- One arm hanging farther away from the body than the other when the arms are allowed to hang loosely by the sides
- Tilting to one side when standing
- A hump on the back at the ribs or near the waist when bending forwards

Parents should report any of these physical signs to their child's doctor. The doctor's physical examination and X-rays will indicate or rule out scoliosis.

Treatment and Care

Sometimes the only treatment needed for scoliosis is to do exercises that stretch the spine and strengthen the muscles of the trunk. In some cases, though, other treatments are necessary to prevent heart and lung problems or back pain later in life. There are several treatment options:

- Wearing a moulded body brace, hidden by clothing, is the most conservative approach. This brace is typically worn most of the day and night for several years. Because the spine grows rapidly during adolescence, wearing a brace at this time can arrest further abnormal curving.
- Surgery to straighten the spine is a more radical alternative, used when the spine is severely curved. A thin steel rod is implanted alongside the spine.

In most instances, scoliosis can be sufficiently treated so that the adolescent doesn't suffer any complications as an adult.

SICKLE-CELL ANAEMIA

If you're an Afro-Caribbean, you will probably know about sickle-cell anaemia. In the UK, about one in 100 black people of West African origin and one in 200 of West Indian origin suffer from sickle-cell anaemia. About one in 10 black people carries the gene for the sickle-cell trait (i.e., they have the ability to produce children with sickle-cell anaemia but have no symptoms of the disease). If both parents carry the trait, the risk of having a child with sickle-cell anaemia is one in four.

Red blood cells are normally round. In sickle-cell anaemia, the red blood cells take on a sickle-cell shape. This makes the blood thicker and affects the red blood cells' ability to carry oxygen to the body's tissues. The disease usually doesn't become apparent until the end of the child's first year. As many as one out of four affected children will die, usually before they're five years old.

Signs and Symptoms

A blood test can detect sickle-cell anaemia, but signs and symptoms include the following:

- Pain, ranging from mild to severe, in the chest, joints, back or abdomen
- Swollen hands and feet
- Jaundice
- Repeated infections, particularly pneumonia or meningitis
- Kidney failure
- Gallstones (at an early age)
- Strokes (at an early age)

Treatment, Care and Prevention

At present there are no drugs that effectively treat sickle-cell anaemia. At best, treatment is geared towards preventing complications. Painful episodes are treated with painkillers, fluids and oxygen, and antibiotics if necessary. The diet is supplemented with folate. Because people with sickle-cell anaemia are prone to developing pneumonia, they should be vaccinated against pneumococci bacteria.

The only possible way to prevent sickle-cell anaemia and to avoid giving birth to children with the disease is to find out whether or not you carry the genes for the disease before you get pregnant. Afro-Caribbean couples should have a blood test to determine if either one is a carrier. After conception, sickle-cell anaemia can be diagnosed by chorionic villus sampling or amniocentesis.

STROKE

Strokes (also called cerebrovascular accidents) are one of the leading causes of death in developed countries. A stroke can be caused by lack of blood (and therefore lack of oxygen) to the brain, usually due to either atherosclerosis or rupture of a blood vessel in the brain. In either case, the end result is brain damage (and possible death). Persons who suffer from both high blood pressure and hardening of the arteries are most susceptible to having a stroke. A stroke can happen suddenly, but it often follows many years in which fatty deposits slowly build up inside the blood vessels.

Some people experience a temporary mini-stroke, or a transient ischaemic attack (TIA). The symptoms mimic a stroke (see Signs and Symptoms) but clear within 24 hours. TIAs are a warning that a real stroke may follow.

Prevention

Measures can be taken to prevent a stroke. Here's what to do to reduce your risks:
- Control your blood pressure. Have it checked regularly and, if necessary, take medication prescribed by your doctor.
- Reduce blood levels of cholesterol to below 5.2 mmol/l (measured by a blood test).
- Get regular exercise.
- Keep your weight down.
- Don't smoke.
- Keep blood-sugar levels under control if you're diabetic.
- Drink alcohol in moderation.
- If you take oral contraceptive pills, don't smoke.
- Learn to manage stress.
- Ask your doctor about taking low-dose aspirin.

Signs and Symptoms

To minimize the damage of a stroke, it's important to know the warning signals of a stroke and get immediate medical attention. To help you remember what to look out for, the initials of the signs and symptoms spell DANGER.
- **D**izziness
- **A**bsent-mindedness, or temporary loss of memory or mental ability
- **N**umbness or weakness in the face, arm or leg
- **G**arbled speech
- **E**ye problems, including temporary loss of sight in one eye or double vision
- **R**ecent onset of severe headaches

Treatment and Care

Tests can be done to locate the obstruction of blood flow to the brain. The doctor may then prescribe appropriate medicines and/or surgery.

When an actual stroke occurs, it is crucial to get immediate treatment. Treatment often includes:

• Medications that reduce brain-tissue swelling, control blood pressure and inhibit the normal clotting of the blood or prevent existing clots from getting bigger
• Surgery if warranted
• Rehabilitation, as needed, by speech therapists, physiotherapists and occupational therapists

THYROID PROBLEMS

The thyroid is a small, butterfly-shaped gland located just in front of the windpipe (trachea) in your throat. Its normal function is to produce thyroxine, a hormone that influences a variety of metabolic processes in the body. These include converting food to energy, regulating growth and fertility and maintaining body temperature. Problems occur when the gland is overactive (hyperthyroidism), when it produces too much hormone, or underactive (hypothyroidism), when it produces too little hormone.

Signs and Symptoms

Overactivity of the thyroid gland (two common forms of which are Graves disease and toxic multi-nodular goitre) occurs when the thyroid produces too much thyroid hormone. Some signs and symptoms are:

• Tremors
• Weakness
• Diarrhoea
• Heart palpitations
• Heat intolerance
• Unexplained weight loss
• Fine hair (or hair loss)
• Rapid pulse
• Nervousness
• Bulging eyes
• Enlarged thyroid gland
• Shortened menstrual periods

Underactivity of the thyroid gland occurs when the thyroid gland does not make enough thyroid hormone to meet the body's needs. Some signs and symptoms are:

• Fatigue and excessive sleeping
• Dry, pale skin
• Deepening of the voice
• Weight gain
• Dry hair that tends to fall out
• Decrease in appetite
• Frequently feeling cold
• Puffy face (especially around the eyes)
• Heavy and/or irregular menstrual periods
• Poor memory
• Constipation
• Enlarged thyroid gland (in some cases)

Treatment, Care and Prevention

Treatment for thyroid problems depends on which condition is present. An underactive thyroid gland is generally treated with medicine to supplement thyroid hormones. A person may require lifelong supplementation and follow-up care to monitor treatment.

Treatment of an overactive thyroid gland varies with the cause, but generally involves one or more of the following:

- Surgical removal of part or all of the thyroid
- Radioactive iodine
- Medicine to stop overproduction of thyroid hormones

Surgical removal and radioactive iodine treatments frequently result in the need to take thyroid supplementation thereafter.

SECTION 3
EMERGENCY PROCEDURES
AND CONDITIONS

ABOUT THIS SECTION

This section contains information that can help you deal with several emergency situations.

- Chapter 14 provides information and drawings to illustrate first aid for choking. You should take a first aid course to learn how to do these procedures and cardiopulmonary resuscitation (CPR) correctly. Doing them incorrectly or inappropriately can cause serious damage.
- Chapter 15 presents six conditions for which emergency care and/or first aid is vital. Read about any emergency condition, and ask yourself the 'Questions to Ask'. Start at the top of the flowchart and answer yes or no to each question. Follow the arrows until you get to one of these answers:
- Seek Emergency Care
- See Doctor
- Call Doctor
- Provide Self-Care

In addition, 'Provide First Aid Procedures for Non-Emergencies' is sometimes given as an answer. A list of first aid procedures for these non-emergencies is provided.

The 'Seek Emergency Care' symbol may direct you to do one of the following:

- Perform CPR if trained (training is available through your local branch of the Red Cross or St John's Ambulance), artificial ventilation, or the Heimlich manoeuvre.
- Give first aid before emergency care. A list of first aid procedures is given.
- Give an injection from, and follow other instructions in, the emergency kit that some highly allergic people carry with them.

If you are alone with a victim, you may need to start first aid before you seek emergency care (as is the case with CPR, artificial ventilation and the Heimlich manoeuvre), but you should yell for help. If you are not alone, let the person who is best trained to give first aid stay with and help the victim. Get someone else to seek emergency care.

When you see the phrase 'And perform first aid before Emergency Care', seek emergency care first and then do the first aid measures listed while you wait for emergency care.

CHAPTER 14
EMERGENCY PROCEDURES

FIRST AID FOR CHOKING

Obstructed Airway: Conscious Adult

Determine if the victim is able to speak or cough, by asking 'Are you choking?' A typical distress signal of choking is clutching the neck between thumb and index finger.

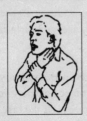

Back Slap

Encourage the victim to cough up the obstruction. If this fails, bend the victim over and give him or her a slap between the shoulder blades. Only if back slapping fails, should you perform an abdominal thrust or a chest thrust (see below).

Abdominal Thrust

Perform the Heimlich manoeuvre until the foreign body is expelled or the victim becomes unconscious. Stand behind the victim and wrap your arms around his or her waist. Press your fist into the victim's abdomen with quick inward and upward thrusts. *Note: You can cause serious damage to the underlying organs if you perform this technique incorrectly.*

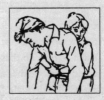

Chest Thrust

For victims who are in advanced pregnancy or who are obese:

Chest thrusts: Stand behind the victim and place your arms under his or her armpits to encircle the chest. Press with quick backward thrusts. *Note: You can cause serious damage to the underlying organs if you perform this technique incorrectly.*

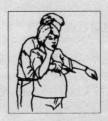

Obstructed Airway:
If Victim Is or Becomes
Unconscious

 Dial 999 – Ask for an emergency ambulance.

 Check for foreign body – Sweep deeply into mouth with hooked finger to remove foreign body.

 Attempt mouth-to-mouth ventilation – Open airway. Try to give two breaths. If needed, reposition the head and try again.

If the airway is obstructed, perform the Heimlich manoeuvre. Kneel astride the victim's thighs. Place the heel of one of your hands on the victim's abdomen, in the centre slightly above the navel and well below the lowest part of the breastbone. Place your other hand on top of the first. Press into the abdomen with up to four quick upward thrusts.

Repeat the following steps until successful, alternating the manoeuvres in rapid sequence:

• Finger sweep of airway
• Mouth-to-mouth ventilation
• Abdominal thrusts

CHAPTER 15
EMERGENCY CONDITIONS

ACCIDENTAL POISONING AND POISONING FIRST AID

Each year millions of cases of accidental poisoning occur. Most of the victims are children, particularly those between one and six years old.

The most common poisons include:
- Medicines (e.g., aspirin, tranquillizers, sleeping pills)
- Household cleaners (e.g., bleach, dishwasher detergent, floor and furniture polishes and waxes, drain cleaners)
- Ammonia
- Insecticides and rat poison
- Vitamins and iron tablets
- Alcoholic beverages
- Hair dye, mouthwash, iodine and mothballs
- Some indoor plants
- Some outdoor plants and berries
- Petrol, antifreeze, oil and other chemicals for the car
- Lighter fluid
- Paint thinner

Most of the damage done by accidental poisons occurs from swallowing. Caustic substances such as drain cleaners quickly destroy tissue as they slide down the throat. Some substances that are toxic can cause serious medical problems when they are inhaled or absorbed through the skin. Some examples are:
- Petrol
- Car exhaust
- Formaldehyde and other chemicals
- Model aeroplane glue

Prevention

To prevent poisoning:
- Keep all potentially poisonous products out of children's reach. Better yet, keep the products locked up.
- Buy and install easy-to-attach, plastic, childproof latches on cupboard doors.
- Do not store hazardous materials or medications in food containers. It's best to keep these items in their original containers, out of reach and out of sight.
- Place plants where children cannot reach a leaf or berry for tasting.
- Store all medications and vitamins in containers with child-resistant tops. Vitamins with iron can be deadly to a small child.
- Read warning labels on pesticides, household cleaners and other potentially poisonous products so you know what to do in the event of an accidental poisoning. Some label instructions may be outdated, so always contact your doctor or local hospital

Accident and Emergency Department if poisoning occurs.

- Flush unused medications down the toilet and rinse the containers before discarding them.
- Teach your child never to touch anything with a skull and crossbones or an orange X hazardous chemical sign on it. These are standard symbols for a poisonous product.
- Never refer to medications or vitamins as 'sweets' in front of a child.
- Wear protective clothing, masks and gloves when using chemicals that could cause harm if inhaled or absorbed by the skin.
- Use potentially dangerous volatile substances only in areas that are well-ventilated. Product labels tell you if ventilation is necessary.

If you are involved with an accidental poisoning, immediately contact your doctor or the local Accident and Emergency Department. Be prepared to give them as much information as possible. This includes:

- The name of the substance taken
- The amount
- The list of ingredients on the product label
- Information about the person who took the poison:
  - His or her age, gender and weight
  - How he or she is feeling and reacting
  - Any medical problems he or she has

If you accompany the victim to hospital, always take the original poison container with you.

Questions to Ask

Is the person not breathing, and does he or she have no pulse? **YES**

 NO

Perform CPR if trained.

Is the person not breathing, but he or she has a pulse? **YES**

 NO

Is the person unconscious or having convulsions? **YES**

 NO

And give first aid before Emergency Care:
Lie the victim down on his or her left side and check airway, breathing and pulse often before Emergency Care. If trained, perform CPR or mouth-to-mouth ventilation if needed.

Has any substance been swallowed, inhaled or absorbed by the skin that:

- Has a 'harmful or fatal if swallowed' warning on the label
- A skull and crossbones or an orange X on the container
- You are unsure whether or not it is poisonous

YES

 NO

And call 999. Remain calm.

223

BREATHING DIFFICULTIES

Allergies and asthma can cause severe breathing difficulties during an attack. Many other people suffer from breathing difficulties due to smog and air polluted by industry, traffic and cigarette smoke.

People who are very allergic to some types of shellfish, nuts, medications and insect bites can also suffer breathing difficulties as part of a severe allergic reaction called anaphylactic shock. This reaction begins within minutes of exposure to the substance causing the allergy. During this type of allergic reaction, the airways narrow, making it difficult to breathe. Soon the heartbeat races and blood pressure drops. Anaphylactic shock can kill if a person is not treated within 15 minutes.

Some types of severe breathing difficulties may require emergency care. In children they include:
• Wheezing
• Croup
• Epiglottitis (inflammation of the flap at the back of the throat that closes off the windpipe during swallowing)

Breathing difficulties in children and adults that may require emergency care include:
• Severe allergic reactions
• A face, head, nose or lung injury
• Carbon monoxide poisoning
• Chemical burns in the air passages
• Choking
• Drug overdose
• Poisoning
• Asthma
• Bronchitis and pneumonia

In adults they include:
• Emphysema
• Congestive heart failure
• Heart attack
• Blood clot in lungs

Prevention

• Avoid allergic substances or agents that induce asthma, if you have it.
• Do not walk, run or jog on roads with heavy traffic.
• If you have a gas boiler or fire, have it checked periodically for safety.
• Never leave your car running in a closed garage.
• Make sure immunizations against childhood diseases are up-to-date.
• If you smoke, stop.
• Keep small objects a child could choke on out of reach and do not give chewing gum, bubble gum, nuts, boiled sweets or popcorn to children under five years old.
• Lock up all medications and poisonous substances so small children can't get to them.

Questions to Ask

Has breathing stopped and is there no pulse? **YES**

NO

And perform CPR if trained.

Has breathing stopped, but there is a pulse? **YES**

NO

And perform Rescue Breathing.

Has breathing stopped due to choking on a swallowed object? **YES**

NO

And perform Heimlich Manoeuvre. (See 'First Aid for Choking' on page 220.)

Are there signs of anaphylactic shock:
- Difficulty in breathing
- Swollen tongue, eyes or face
- Unconsciousness
- Difficulty in swallowing
- Dizziness, weakness
- Pounding heart
- Itching, hives

YES

NO

Inject the substance from the emergency kit that some very allergic people carry with them, if available. Follow all the instructions in the kit.

flowchart continued in next column

Are any of these problems present with difficulty in breathing:
- Signs of a heart attack (e.g., chest pain, pressure or tightness, pain that spreads to the arm, neck or jaw, irregular pulse)
- Serious injury to the face, head or chest
- Signs of a stroke (e.g., blurred or double vision, slurred speech, one-sided body weakness or paralysis)
- Signs of drug overdose (e.g., behaving as though drunk, slurred speech, slow or rapid pulse, heavy sweating, enlarged or very small eye pupils)

YES

NO

Is it so hard to breathe that you or someone else can't talk (say four or five words between breaths) and/or is there wheezing that doesn't go away? **YES**

NO

Is bloody phlegm being coughed up? **YES**

NO

flowchart continued on next page

In a baby does the difficulty in breathing occur with a cough and make the baby unable to eat or take a bottle? **YES**

NO

Is there:
• Breathlessness at night or at rest
• Pink or frothy phlegm being coughed up and/or
• A high fever along with the rapid and laboured breathing

YES

NO

Is greenish-yellow or grey phlegm being coughed up? **YES**

NO

Self-Care Procedures

For people affected by air pollution or pollen:
• Don't smoke. Avoid second-hand smoke. *Note: This applies to anyone with breathing difficulties.*
• Wear a face mask that covers the nose and mouth (e.g., when cycling in heavy traffic).

For people allergic to moulds, breathing problems can be avoided or lessened if you:
• Do not rake leaves that have been on the ground for a while. Moulds and mildew grow on leaves after they've been on the ground for a few days.
• Get rid of house plants.

If you or anyone in your family has severe allergies, it is a good idea to wear a medical identification tag such as those available from the Medic-Alert Foundation (0171 833 3034).

See Chapter 2 for Self-Care Procedures for asthma, bronchitis, common cold, coughs and flu. See Chapter 8 for Self-Care Procedures for croup.

DRUG OVERDOSE

Drug overdoses can be accidental or intentional. The amount of a drug needed to cause problems varies with the type of drug and the person taking it. Overdoses from prescription and over-the-counter (OTC) medicines, 'street' drugs and/or alcohol can be life-threatening. Know, too, that mixing certain medications or 'street' drugs with alcohol can also kill.

Physical symptoms of a drug overdose vary with the type of drug(s) taken. They include:
• Abnormal breathing
• Slurred speech
• Lack of coordination
• Slow or rapid pulse
• Low or elevated body temperature
• Enlarged or small eye pupils
• Reddish face
• Heavy sweating
• Delusions and/or hallucinations
• Drowsiness, sleep which may lead to coma

Parents need to watch for signs of illegal drug and alcohol use in their children. Morning hangovers, the smell of alcohol and red streaks in the whites of the eyes are obvious signs of alcohol use. Items such as pipes, rolling papers, eye droppers and butane lighters may be the first telling clues that someone is abusing drugs. Other clues are behaviour changes such as:

- Lack of appetite
- Insomnia
- Hostility
- Mental confusion
- Depression
- Mood swings
- Secretive behaviour
- Social isolation
- Hallucinations
- Deep sleep

Prevention

Accidental overdoses of prescription and over-the-counter drugs may be prevented by asking your doctor or pharmacist:

- What is the medication and why is it being prescribed?
- How and when should the medication be taken and for how long? (Follow the instructions exactly as given.)
- Can the medication be taken with other medicines or alcohol, or should it not be?
- Are there any foods to avoid while taking this medication?
- What are the possible side effects?
- What are the symptoms of an overdose and what should be done if it occurs?

- Should any activities be avoided (e.g., operating heavy machinery, driving and exposure to sun)?
- Should the medicine still be taken even if there is a preexisting medical condition?

Medication overdoses can be avoided by observing the following:
- Never take a medicine prescribed for someone else.
- Never give or take medication in the dark. Before each dose, always read the label on the bottle to be certain it is the correct medication.
- Always tell the doctor of any previous side effects or adverse reactions to medications as well as new and unusual symptoms that occur after taking the current medicine.
- Always store medications in the original containers with childproof lids and place them on high shelves, out of a child's reach, or in locked cupboards.
- Take the prescribed dose, not more.

Illicit drug use among children can be discouraged by observing the following:
- Set a good example for your children by not using drugs yourself.
- Teach your child to say no to drugs and alcohol. Explain the dangers of drug use, including the risk of AIDS.
- Get to know your children's friends and their parents.
- Know where your children are and who they are with.
- Listen to your children and help them express their feelings and fears.
- Encourage your children to engage in healthy activities such as sports,

community-based youth programmes and volunteer work.
- Learn to recognize the signs of drug and alcohol abuse.

Questions to Ask

Is the person not breathing and has no pulse? YES

NO

And perform CPR if trained.

Is the person not breathing, but has a pulse? YES

NO

And perform mouth-to-mouth ventilation.

Is the person unconscious? YES

NO

And give first aid before Emergency Care:
Lie the victim down on his or her left side and check airway, breathing and pulse often before Emergency Care. Perform CPR if trained or Rescue Breathing as needed.

Is the person hallucinating, confused, having convulsions, breathing slowly and shallowly and/or slurring words? YES

NO

flowchart continued in next column

Do you suspect the person has taken an overdose of drugs? YES

NO

See 'Accidental Poisoning and Poisoning First Aid' on page 222.

Is the person's personality suddenly hostile, violent and aggressive? YES

NO

Note: Use caution. Protect yourself. Do not turn your back to the victim or move suddenly in front of him or her. If you can, see that the victim does not harm you, himself or herself. Remember, the victim is under the influence of a drug. Call the police to assist you if you cannot handle the situation. Leave and find a safe place to stay until the police arrive.

Have you or someone else accidentally taken more than the prescribed dose of a prescription or over-the-counter medicine? YES

228

EYE INJURIES

There are many causes of eye injuries. These include:
- Physical blow to the eye
- Caustic chemicals, such as bleach and acids, which can burn eye tissue and permanently damage the eyes
- A grain of sand, fleck of paint, sliver of metal or splinter of wood, which can scratch the cornea and induce infection
- Excessive exposure to the sun, very low humidity or a strong wind, which may dry the eyes so much they feel like sandpaper rubbing against your lids
- Insect bites

Prevention

- Wear protective plastic glasses during sports and other potentially dangerous activities.
- Be careful when using caustic chemicals. Wear rubber gloves and protective glasses. Don't rub your eyes if you've touched caustic chemicals. Wash your hands. Turn your head away from chemical vapours so as not to let any get into your eyes.
- Don't allow a child to stick his or her head out of the window of a moving vehicle. Sand, insects and other flying objects can strike the eye like a flying missile, irritating or damaging the cornea.
- Use artificial teardrops if recommended by your doctor.
- Never stare directly at the sun, especially during a solar eclipse.
- Wear sunglasses that block UV rays whenever you're in the sun.

All eye injuries should be taken seriously and all should be checked by a physician.

Questions to Ask

 Is there a foreign body sticking into the eye? **YES**

NO

And perform first aid procedures before Emergency Care:
- Do not try to remove object.
- Do not press on, touch or rub eye(s).
- Wash hands with soap and water.
- Lightly cover the affected eye with an eyepad or gauze, held in place with tape.
- Also, if possible, lightly cover the unaffected eye, as this will help keep the affected eye from moving. *Note: If you are alone, phone or yell for help. Do not cover the unaffected eye, but try to keep it from moving.*

 Is there a severe blow to the eye, with or without a broken bone of the face? **YES**

NO

flowchart continued on next page

And perform first aid
procedures before
Emergency Care:
• Close the eye.
• Put a cold compress over
the injured area, not directly
on, the eye. You can use ice
(in a plastic bag or wrapped in
a cloth) or a bag of frozen
vegetables.
• Do not use firm pressure.
• Get the victim to sit still
with his or her eyes closed if
possible.
*Note: If you are alone, phone or
yell for help.*

Is there a cut to the eye
or eyelid, or did the
injury occur when you
were hammering metal
or stone even if there is
no visible foreign body in
the eye?

And perform first aid
procedures before
Emergency Care:
• Lightly cover both the
victim's eyes with a sterile
cloth or pad, held in place
with tape.
• Get the victim to sit still
with his or her eyes closed if
possible.
*Note: If you are alone, phone or
yell for help. Do not cover the
unaffected eye but try to keep it
from moving.*

Have harmful chemicals
got into the eye(s)?

*Flush the eye(s) with water
immediately!* Then Seek
Emergency Care

How to flush the eyes with
water:
• Get the victim to lie down
and turn his or her head to
the side with the affected eye
lower than the other eye.
• Hold the affected eye open
with your thumb and
forefinger.
• Pour large quantities of
warm water, not hot, from a
clean pitcher or other clean
container, over the entire eye
starting at the inside corner
and downwards to the
outside corner. This lets the
water drain away from the
body and keeps it from
getting in the other eye.
Continue pouring the water
for at least 10 minutes – 30
minutes is better.
• Loosely bandage the eye
with sterile cloth and tape.
• Do not touch the eye.
• If both eyes are affected,
pour water over both eyes at
the same time or quickly
alternate the above
procedure from one eye to
the other.

• Or place the victim's face in a sink or container filled with warm water. Get the person to move his or her eyelids up and down. *Note: Do this procedure if you are alone.*
• You can also use commercial eye solutions, if available.

Has a bee sting or insect bite to the eye caused a severe allergic reaction with these symptoms:
• Wheezing, shortness of breath and breathing difficulties
• Severe swelling the eye and in other parts of the body such as the tongue, lips and throat
• Bluish lips and skin
• Collapse

YES

NO

Give an injection and follow other instructions from an emergency insect kit, if available.
Note: You can get this kit only with a doctor's prescription.

Do any of these problems occur after an eye injury:
• Blurred or double vision
• Blood in the pupil

YES

NO

Does eye pain last longer than two days?

YES

NO

First Aid Procedures for Non-Emergencies:

To remove a foreign object in the eye:
• Wash your hands.
• Twist a piece of tissue, moisten the tip with tap water, not saliva, and gently try to touch the speck with the tip. As you carefully pass the tissue over the speck, it should cling to the tip.
• If the foreign object is under the upper lid, look down and pull the upper lid away from the eyeball by gently grabbing the eyelashes. Try to touch the debris with the tip of a moistened tissue until it is caught on the tissue.
• Do not rub the eye. And never use tweezers or anything sharp to remove a foreign object. Doing so can scratch the cornea.
• Gently wash the eye with cool water.
• Cover the eye with a patch and leave this in position for at least 24 hours. This helps to relieve the pain.

To treat a black eye from a minor injury:
• Immediately put a cold compress over the injured area. This helps to slow bleeding under the skin and lessens swelling and discoloration.
• Take aspirin or ibuprofen for the pain and inflammation. Paracetamol will help the pain, but not the inflammation.
Note: Do not give aspirin, or any medication containing salicylates, to children under 12 years of age, due to its association with Reye's syndrome, a potentially fatal condition.
• Later, put a warm compress over the injured area.

231

- Seek medical attention if these measures do not help.

To ease the discomfort of dry eyes:
- Try an over-the-counter artificial tear product (ask your pharmacist). Check the label. If there are no preservatives, keep the solution refrigerated. Always wash your hands before putting drops in the eyes.

To ease the discomfort of an insect bite that has not caused a severe allergic reaction:
- Gently wash the eye(s) with warm water.
- Ask your doctor or pharmacist whether or not you should take an antihistamine and ask him or her to recommend one.

HEAT EXHAUSTION AND HEAT STROKE

Perspiration acts like natural air-conditioning. As perspiration evaporates from our skin, it cools us off, especially on hot, sweltering days. But, like a room air conditioner, our personal cooling system can fail if we over-exert ourselves on hot and humid days. When this happens, our body heat climbs to dangerous levels, causing heat exhaustion or life-threatening heat stroke.

Heat exhaustion takes time to develop. Fluids and salt so vital for maintaining good health are lost as children and adults perspire heavily during exercise or other strenuous activity. That's why it is

very important to drink plenty of liquids before, during and after exercise in hot weather. Strange as it seems, people suffering from heat exhaustion have low, normal or only slightly raised body temperatures.

Signs and symptoms of heat exhaustion include:
- Cool, clammy, pale skin
- Sweating
- Dry mouth
- Fatigue, weakness
- Dizziness
- Headache
- Nausea, sometimes vomiting
- Muscle cramps
- Weak and rapid pulse

Heat stroke, unlike heat exhaustion, strikes suddenly, with little warning. When the body's cooling system fails, the body's temperature rapidly rises, creating an emergency condition.

Signs of heat stroke include:
- Very high temperature: 40°C (104°F) or higher
- Hot, dry, red skin
- No sweating
- Deep breathing and fast pulse, followed by shallow breathing and weak pulse
- Dilated pupils
- Confusion, delirium, hallucinations
- Convulsions
- Loss of consciousness

Chronic medical conditions such as diabetes, use of alcohol, and vomiting or diarrhoea can put children and adults at risk of heat stroke during very hot weather. Heat stroke in children is not only due to high temperatures and humidity, but also to not drinking enough fluids.

Prevention

Heat exhaustion and heat stroke can be prevented by following this advice:
- Do not stay in or leave anyone in closed, parked cars during hot weather.
- Take caution when you must be in the sun. At the first signs of heat exhaustion, get out of the sun or your body temperature will continue to rise.
- Do not exercise vigorously during the hottest times of the day. Instead, run, jog or exercise closer to sunrise or sunset. If the outside temperature is 28°C (82°F) or above and the humidity is high, consider shortening your activity session.
- Wear light, loose-fitting clothing (preferably cotton), so sweat can evaporate. Also wear a well-ventilated, wide-brimmed hat.
- Drink lots of liquids, especially if your urine is a very dark yellow or amber, to replace the fluids lost from perspiring. Thirst is not a reliable sign that your body needs fluids. When you exercise, it is better to sip rather than gulp drinks.
- Drink water or water with salt added if you sweat a lot. (Use $^1/_2$ teaspoon salt in about half a litre/one pint of water.) Isotonic sport drinks are good too.
- If you feel very hot, try to cool off by opening a window, using a fan or turning on an air conditioner.

- Limit your stay in hot baths or heated jacuzzis to 15 minutes. Never use them when you are alone.
- Do not drink alcohol or drinks with caffeine because they speed up fluid loss.
- Stay out of the sun if you are taking diuretics, mood-altering drugs or antispasmodic medications. Ask your doctor which ones are safe.
- Do not cover a baby with blankets or dress him or her in thick clothing. Infants don't tolerate heat well because their sweat glands are not well developed.
- Some people perspire more than others. Those who do should drink as much fluid as they can during hot, humid days.
- Know the signs of heat stroke and heat exhaustion and don't ignore them.

Questions to Ask

Are any signs of heat stroke present:
- Body temperature 40°C (104°F) or higher
- Skin that is red, dry and/or hot
- Pulse that is rapid and then gets weak
- No sweating
- Confusion, hallucinations or loss of consciousness or convulsions

flowchart continued on next page

Give first aid for heat stroke before Emergency Care:
• Do CPR (if trained) if the person is not breathing and has no pulse.
• Do mouth-to-mouth ventilation if the victim is not breathing, but does have a pulse.

Until emergency care arrives, it is important to lower the body temperature.

To do this:
• Move the victim to a cool place indoors or under a shady tree. Place the feet higher than the head.
• Remove the clothing and either wrap the victim in a cold, wet sheet; sponge the victim with towels or sheets that are soaked in very cold water; or spray the victim with cool water. Fan the victim. If using an electric fan, take care. Make sure your hands are dry when you plug the fan in and turn it on. Keep the victim and all wet items far enough away from the fan so as not to cause electric shock.
• Put ice packs or cold compresses to the neck, under the armpits and to the groin area.
• Immerse a child in cold water if he or she is unconscious.

• Place the person in the recovery position once his or her temperature reaches 101°F

To do this:
• Kneel at the side of the person. Straighten the victim's arm that is closest to you and raise it above his or her head.
• Cross their other arm over their chest. Bend the victim's far leg and cross it over their near leg.
• Hold the victim's clothing at the hip and gently pull him or her towards you, moving the head with the body.
• Bend the victim's upper arm and leg until each forms a right angle to the body.
• Cover the victim with a wet sheet. If the temperature starts to climb, repeat all of the above.
• Give as much cold water as the person can drink until he or she feels better.

Is the person too dizzy or weak to stand or does he or she have persistent vomiting? YES

 NO

Perform first aid for heat stroke before Emergency Care (see page 234).

flowchart conrinued on next page

Are two or more of these signs of heat exhaustion present:
- Pale, cool and clammy skin
- Sweating
- Dry mouth
- Dizziness
- Fatigue and weakness
- Headache
- Nausea, vomiting
- Weak and rapid pulse
- Muscle cramps

YES

NO

And perform first aid procedures for heat exhaustion.

First Aid Procedures for Heat Exhaustion:

(These apply to you or anyone else who has heat exhaustion symptoms.)
- Move to a cool place indoors or in the shade.
- Loosen clothing.
- Take fluids such as cool or cold water. If available, add $1/2$ teaspoon of salt to about half a litre (one pint) of water and sip it, or drink isotonic sport drinks.
- Eat salty foods like crisps, if tolerated.
- Lie down in a cool, breezy place.

NECK AND SPINE INJURIES

Anything that puts too much pressure or force on the neck or back can result in a neck and/or spinal injury. Suspect a neck injury, too, if a head injury has occurred. Common causes are:
- Accidents involving cars, motorcycles, toboggans, roller blades and the like
- Falls, especially from high places
- Diving mishaps (e.g., diving into water that is too shallow)
- A hard blow to the neck or back while playing a contact sport such as rugby
- Violent acts (e.g., a gunshot wound that penetrates the head, neck or trunk)

Some neck and spinal injuries can be serious because of their potential for causing paralysis. These need emergency medical care. Others (e.g., whiplash injuries) may cause only temporary, minor problems.

A mild whiplash injury typically causes neck pain and stiffness the following day. Some people, though, have trouble raising their heads off the pillow the next morning. Physiotherapy and a collar to support the neck are the most common types of treatment. In many cases it takes three to four months for all the symptoms to disappear.

Prevention

- Use padded head-rests in your car to prevent whiplash injuries.
- Drive carefully.

- Wear seatbelts.
- Buckle children into approved car seats appropriate for their ages.
- Wear a helmet whenever riding bicycles or motorcycles or when roller-skating or roller-blading.
- Wear the recommended safety equipment for contact sports.
- Be careful when jumping up and down on a trampoline, climbing a ladder or checking a roof.
- Check the depth before diving into water. Do not dive into water that is less that 2.7 m (9 ft) deep.

Note: If you suspect a neck or back injury in you or someone else, it is imperative to keep the neck and/or back perfectly still until emergency help arrives. Do not move someone with a suspected neck or spine injury unless the person must be moved because his or her safety is in danger. Any movement of the head, neck or back could result in paralysis or death. Immobilize the neck by holding the head, neck and shoulders perfectly still. Use both hands, one on each side of the head.

Questions to Ask

Is the injured person not breathing and has no pulse? YES

 NO

And perform CPR if trained, but without moving the neck or spine. Do not tilt the head back or move the head or neck. Instead, pull the lower jaw (chin) forward to open the airway.

Is the injured person not breathing, but has a pulse? YES

NO

And perform mouth-to-mouth ventilation without moving the neck or spine, but do not tilt the head back or move the head or neck. Instead, pull the lower jaw (chin) forward to open the airway.

Additional first aid procedures before Emergency Care:
• Tell the victim to lie still and not move his or her head, neck, back, etc.
• Immobilize the neck and/or spine. Place rolled towels, articles of clothing, etc. on both sides of the neck and/or body. Tie and wrap in place, but don't interfere with the victim's breathing. If necessary, use both of your hands, one on each side of the victim's head, to keep the head from moving.

Do not move anyone with a suspected neck or spinal injury unless they are in danger from fire or some other hazard. If a victim must be moved, follow the above procedures and:

- Select a stretcher, door or other rigid board.
- Use several people to lift and move the injured person gently onto the board, being very careful to align the head and neck in a straight line with the spine. The head should not rotate or bend forward or backward.
- Make sure one person uses both of his or her hands, one on each side of the victim's head, to keep the head from moving. If you can, immobilize the neck and/or spine by placing rolled towels, articles of clothing, etc. on both sides of the neck and/or body. Tie and wrap them in place, but don't interfere with the victim's breathing.

If you suspect someone has injured his or her neck in a diving or other water accident:
- Protect the neck and/or spine from bending or twisting. Place your hands on both sides of his or her neck and keep in place until help arrives.
- If the victim is still in the water, help him or her to float until a rigid board can be slipped under his or her head and body, at least as far down as the buttocks.
- If no board is available, several people should take the victim out of the water, supporting his or her head

and body as one unit, making sure the head does not rotate or bend in any direction.

Does the injured person have any of these signs or symptoms:
- Paralysis
- Inability to open and close his or her fingers or move his or her toes
- Feelings of numbness in the legs, arms, shoulders or any other part of the body
- Appearance that the head, neck or back is in an odd position

 NO

Are any of these present following a recent injury to the neck and/or spine that did not get treated with emergency care at the time of the injury?
- Severe pain
- Numbness, tingling or weakness in the face, arms or legs
- Loss of bladder control

 NO

Do you suspect a whiplash injury, or has pain from any injury to the neck or back lasted longer than one week?

 NO

237

Self-Care Procedures

If you suspect a whiplash injury:

- See your doctor as soon as you can so he or she can assess the extent of injury.
- For the first 24 hours, apply ice packs to the injured area for up to 20 minutes an hour.
- To make an ice pack, wrap ice in a facecloth or towel.
- After 24 hours, use ice packs or heat to relieve the pain.
- Take a hot shower for 20 minutes a few times a day. This is a good source of heat to the neck.
- Use a wrapped hot water bottle, heating pad (set on low) or a heat lamp directed to the neck for 10 minutes several times a day.
- Use a cervical pillow or a small rolled towel positioned behind your neck instead of a regular pillow.
- Wrap a folded towel around the neck to help hold the head in one position during the night.
- Take aspirin, paracetamol or ibuprofen for minor pain. *Note: Do not give aspirin, or any medication containing salicylates, to children under 12 years of age, due to its association with Reye's syndrome, a potentially fatal condition.*
- Get plenty of rest, preferably lying down. (When sitting, the neck is still working to support the weight of the head.)

SELF CARE:
USEFUL ADDRESSES & PHONE NUMBERS

AGEING

Age Concern England
Astral House
1268 London Rd
London SW16 4ER
Tel: 0181 6719 8000

Age Concern Cymru
4th floor, Transport House
1 Cathedral Rd
Cardiff CF1 9SD
Tel: 01222 371 566

Age Concern Northern Ireland
3 Lower Crescent
Belfast BT7 1NR
Tel: 01232 245729

Age Concern Scotland
113 Rose St
Edinburgh EH2 3DT
Tel: 0131 220 3345

AIDS

Positively Women
347–349 City Rd
London EC1V 1LR
Tel: 0171 713 0444

Terrence Higgins Trust
52–54 Grays Inn Rd
London WC1X 8JU
Tel: 0171 242 1010

ALCOHOL PROBLEMS

Alcoholics Anonymous
PO Box 1
Stonebow House
Stonebow
York YO1 2NJ
Tel (head office): 01904 644026
See telephone directory for local
numbers.

Alanon Family Groups; Alateen
61 Great Dover St
London SE1 4YF
Tel: 0171 403 0888

ALZHEIMER'S DISEASE

Alzheimer's Disease Society
2nd floor, Gordon House
10 Greencoat Place
London SW1P 1PH
Tel: 0171 306 0606

ARTHRITIS AND RHEUMATISM

Arthritis and Rheumatism Council
for Research
Copeman House
St Mary's Court
St Mary's Gate
Chesterfield S41 7TD
Tel: 01246 558033

Arthritis Care
18 Stephenson Way
London NW1 2HD
Tel: 0800 289170

ASTHMA

National Asthma Campaign
Providence House
Providence Place
London N1 0NT
Tel: 0171 226 2260

BACK PAIN

National Back Pain Association
16 Elmtree Rd
Teddington
Middlesex TW11 8ST
Tel: 0181 977 5474

BEREAVEMENT

Cruse-Bereavement Care
Cruse House
126 Sheen Rd
Richmond
Surrey TW9 1UR
Tel: 0181 940 4818

CANCER

BACUP (British Association of Cancer
United Patients)
3 Bath Place
Rivington St
London EC2A 3JR
Tel: 0800 181199

Breast Cancer Care
Kiln House
210 New King's Rd
London SW6 4NZ
Tel: 01500 245345

Cancer Care Society
21 Zetland Rd
Redland
Bristol BS6 7AH
Tel: 0117 942 7419

Cancer Relief Macmillan Fund
15/19 Britten St
London SW3 3TZ
Tel: 0171 351 7811

Leukaemia Care Society
14 Kingfisher Court
Vennybridge
Pinhoe
Exeter EX4 8JN
Tel: 013924 64848

CARING

Black Carers Support Group
Annie Wood Resource Centre
129 Alma Way
Lozells
Birmingham
West Midlands B19 2LS
Tel: 0121 554 7137

Carers National Association
20–25 Glasshouse Yard
London EC1A 4JS
Tel: 0171 490 8818

CYSTIC FIBROSIS

Cystic Fibrosis Trust
Alexandra House
5 Blyth Rd
Bromley
Kent BR1 3RSJ
Tel: 0181 464 7211

DIABETES

British Diabetic Association
10 Queen Anne St
London W1M 0BD
Tel: 0171 323 1531

DIGESTIVE PROBLEMS

British Digestive Foundation
(Publications)
PO Box 251
Edgware
Middlesex HA8 6HG
Tel: 0171 486 0341

DISABILITY

Disability Alliance
Universal House
88 Wentworth St
London E1 7SA
Tel: 0171 247 8776

DRUG PROBLEMS

Release (The National Drugs and Legal
Helpline)
388 Old St
London EC1V 9LT
Tel: 0171 729 9904

EATING DISORDERS

Eating Disorders Association
Sackville Place
44 Magdalen St
Norwich NR3 1JU
Tel: 01603 621414

ECZEMA

National Eczema Society
163 Eversholt St
London NW1 1BU
Tel: 0171 338 4097

ENDOMETRIOSIS

National Endometriosis Society
Suite 50
Westminster Palace Gardens
1/7 Artillery Row
London SW1P 1RL
Tel: 0171 222 2781

EPILEPSY

British Epilepsy Association
Anstey House
40 Hanover Square
Leeds LS3 1BE
Tel: 0345 089599

EYE PROBLEMS

International Glaucoma Association
King's College Hospital
Denmark Hill
London SE5 9RS
Tel: 0171 737 3265

RNIB
(Royal National Institute for the Blind)
224 Great Portland St
London W1N 6AA
Tel: 0171 388 1266

FIRST AID

Red Cross
Contact your local branch for details of
first aid courses

St John's Ambulance
Contact your local branch for details of
first aid courses

HEALTH EDUCATION

Health Education Authority
Hamilton House
Mabledon Place
London WC1H 9TX
Tel: 0171 383 3833

HEARING PROBLEMS

National Deaf Children's Society
15 Dufferin St
London EC1Y 8PD
Tel: 0800 252380

British Deaf Association
38 Victoria Place
Carlisle
Cumbria CA1 1HU
Tel: 01228 48844

RNID
(Royal National Institute for Deaf People)
19–23 Featherstone St
London EC1Y 8SL
Tel: 0171 387 8033
Minicom: 0171296 8001

British Tinnitus Association
14–18 West Bar Green
Sheffield
South Yorkshire S1 2DA
Tel: 0114 2796600

HEART DISEASE

British Heart Foundation
14 Fitzhardinge St
London W1H 4DH
Tel: 0171 935 0185

HERPES

Herpes Association
41 North Road
London N7 9DP
Tel: 0171 609 9061

INCONTINENCE

Association of Continence Advice
2 Doughty St
London WC1N 2PH
Tel: 0171 404 6875

Enuresis Resource and Information
Centre
65 St Michael's Hill
Bristol BS2 8DZ
Tel: 0117 9264920

LUNG PROBLEMS

British Lung Foundation
78 Hatton Garden
London EC1N 8JR
Tel: 0171 831 5831

LUPUS

Lupus UK
1 Eastern Road
Romford
Essex RM1 3NH
Tel: 01708 731251

ME (MYALGIC ENCEPHALOMYELITIS)

ME Association
Stanhope House
High St
Stamford-le-Hope
Essex SS17 0HA
Tel: 01375 361013

MEDIC-ALERT

Medic-Alert Foundation
2 Bridge Wharf
156 Caledonian Rd
London N1 9UU
Tel: 0171 833 3034

MENTAL HEALTH

MIND
(National Association for Mental Health)
Granta House
15–19 Broadway
Stratford
London E15 4BQ
Tel: 0181 519 2122

Samaritans, The
10 The Grove
Slough
Berks SL1 1QP
Tel: 01753 532713 (administration);
0345 909090 (help-line)

MIGRAINE

British Migraine Association
178a High Road
Byfleet
West Byfleet
Surrey KT14 7ED
Tel: 01932 352468

MULTIPLE SCLEROSIS

Multiple Sclerosis Society
25 Effie Rd
London SW6 1EE
Tel: 0171 371 8000

OSTEOPOROSIS

National Osteoporosis Society
PO Box 10
Radstock
Bath BA3 3YB
Tel: 01761 471771

OVERWEIGHT

Weight Watchers UK
Kidwells Park House
Kidwells Park Drive
Maidenhead
Berks SL6 8YT
Tel: 01628 777077

PARKINSON'S DISEASE

Parkinson's Disease Society
22 Upper Woburn Place
London WC1H 0RA
Tel: 0171 383 3513

PREGNANCY

National Childbirth Trust
Alexandra House
Oldham Terrace
London W3 6NH
Tel: 0181 992 8637

SICKLE-CELL DISEASE

Sickle Cell Society
54 Station Rd
Harlesden
London NW10 4UA
Tel: 0181 961 4006

SMOKING

Quitline
Victory House
170 Tottenham Court Rd
London W1P 0HA
Tel: 0171 487 3000

STROKE

Stroke Association
CHSA House
123–127 Whitecross St
London EC1Y 8JJ
Tel: 0171 490 7999

WOMEN'S HEALTH

National Association for Premenstrual
Syndrome
PO Box 72
Sevenoaks
Kent TN13 1XQ
Tel: 01732 741709

Women's Health Concern
(Publications)
Well Wood
North Farm Rd
Tonbridge Wells
Kent
Tel: 0181 780 3007

INDEX